An Autoimmune Food Journey

Welcome
To Your

FLog!

**A 30 Day Food Log For Those Who Want to
Feel Amazing Every Day!**

Angela M. Landeros

ISBN 978-1-959182-06-1 (paperback)
ISBN 978-1-959182-07-8 (digital)

Angela Landeros Heals
818-835-1217

Printed in the United States of America

Special Thanks and Dedication

First, I would like to thank God for standing beside me throughout my entire life. Second, I thank my husband who has had to listen to me for countless hours on what will make the best food journal ever, The FLog! He's had a front row view on how it's changed my health for the better. Thank you to all my volunteer readers who helped edit! A special thanks to Dr. Michael Campbell, DC. for answering my endless functional medicine questions. I am truly blessed to know you. I dedicate this book to all who choose to FLog their lifestyles into shape. You are why I have fought for myself, because I am focused on helping others.

Thank you to all the people and naturopathic doctors I have cited in this book. You are all truly my doctors and supporters, even if you never treated me in your offices. Nevertheless, you are all a part of my treatment! You helped change my perspective on food and whether conquering disease was possible.

Disclaimer:

FLog Contents

Welcome to Your 30 Day FLog!

The FLog is for people who:

Want to feel amazing, regardless of whether they are supreme athletes, regular people, or dealing with health issues. That means *you*! It will help you make the right choices so that you can feel your best every day.

It will give you an opportunity to:

Change your body chemistry by keeping track of what you put in your body. You can improve your immune system, heal your digestive system, strengthen your brain, and reduce inflammation throughout your whole body. Your body is a temple and a functioning super system. Treat it well by eating for its unique needs, while reducing mental and physical stress.

In your FLog you will:

Input your type of sleep, food, liquid intake, exercise, moods and symptoms into your FLog. And yes, even your poop. You will grade yourself on a daily basis according to the foods and liquids you consume and the symptoms you feel afterwards. Eventually you will create a list of substances that have a negative effect on your body, substances you should never eat or come into contact with, and those that you may consume occasionally.

You are on your way to:

Your best self by learning self-discipline and avoiding the instant gratification of eating and drinking things that make you feel good for only a moment but lead to regret once you feel the consequences. The self-destructive habits will slowly disappear from your lifestyle because feeling your best is addictive!

Learn From My Journey

Between each week of logging your data, you will read about my own journey to achieving wellness—the victories, the failures, and how I never gave up. I hope my story will encourage you to keep going and keep healing. I interspersed my story through your FLog pages each week because I want you to focus on your journey but also hope that you will be inspired by mine.

Before you start:

You should take some time before you start The FLog and reflect on the present state of your health, your relationship with food, your overall wellbeing, and why you want to feel better. It is not necessary to write down these feelings, but it may be helpful to put them in the first day's log page under "Notes and Thoughts" and revisit them periodically during your journey. There is no need to pre-set goals and expectations now. Get started, take it one day at a time, and hold yourself accountable.

I wish you success and a long healthy life.

You are worth it!

Follow Angela on social media, we're all in this together.
Instagram: @angela_landeros_heals

WTFLog?

The purpose of The FLog is not to count calories, but rather to keep track of what you put in your body and how those ingredients make you feel. My own journey toward a healthier immune system began with months of questioning why my skin was breaking out in hives and rashes and why I was diagnosed with multiple sclerosis. After listening to my first webinar on auto immunity and naturopathic medicine, I spent two years sifting through my diet trying to eliminate inflammatory foods from my eating habits. It took me another two years to find a diet that suited my unique needs based on what I had learned and by keeping track of how my body reacted to what I put in it. I can't tell you what specific 'diet' is right for you because everyone is different. I *can* tell you what foods to avoid and a general why. Your body is unique, therefore you may find yourself having a negative reaction to certain foods that other people can consume without any issues.

You will find that certain foods cause an immediate reaction, while others have delayed reactions. All of these food groups, including those in the FODMAPs section of this book, may be inflammatory to you. An inflammatory reaction is your body's defensive reaction to a substance. It is the same as when your body fights an infection—your body sees a substance as foreign and reacts.

> *"IA 2010 survey of the Society for Nutrition Therapy and Prevention e.V. reported that 67% of respondents suffer from intermittent or persistent gastrointestinal symptoms including bloating or abdominal pain after eating. An important cause may be food intolerance, which is mediated by the innate immune system. It leads to typical adverse reactions and inflammatory processes. Defense reactions, e.g. of neutrophils, create the basis for micro inflammation and centres of inflammation. The whole system is a very effective first defense strategy against acute infections but chronic activation will lead to health disorders. A study by the University of Pavia in 2011 on 48 patients with gastrointestinal disorders (GI) and 35 patients with skin problems (H) illustrates the influence of incompatible foods in the body: the not tolerated substances were removed from the diet, improved symptoms after 2 months significant at 71% (GI) and 66% (H) of the patients."*

[1] Endnote - *Society for Nutrition Therapy and Prevention*

The FLog's protocol is meant to rebalance your digestive health through the elimination of inflammatory foods and eating a strict diet consisting mainly of organic vegetables, moderate animal proteins, fats, minimal fruits and carbohydrates. Not only can you achieve a more desirable weight by following a non-inflammatory food regime but the improvements in your overall health will be satisfying and will motivate you to continue on the journey to better health, energy, digestion, and even brain function.

Unlike many fad diets, The FLog protocol is not meant to be a short detox or period of elimination after which you return to your old eating habits. It is a lifestyle change, in which every day you will challenge yourself to either stay on the perfect protocol for your particular body or you may make decisions that you will later regret. Your body will give you the answers if you pay attention to the signs. This is your guide to your best self and if you screw up, you can start again the next day. Your diet will change many times in your journey to create your body's perfect food protocol. There is no need to label it, regardless of whether you consider yourself a vegan, Paleolithic, or whether you eat everything in sight. This is your individual journey, but you may find that there are other 'FLoggies' who follow similar regimes who can learn from you and you can learn from them.

Your Superhero Self
Digestive and Immune System

The decisions you make can either help your body or burden your body. Be a superhero and help it out! Let's take a moment to talk about your immune system.

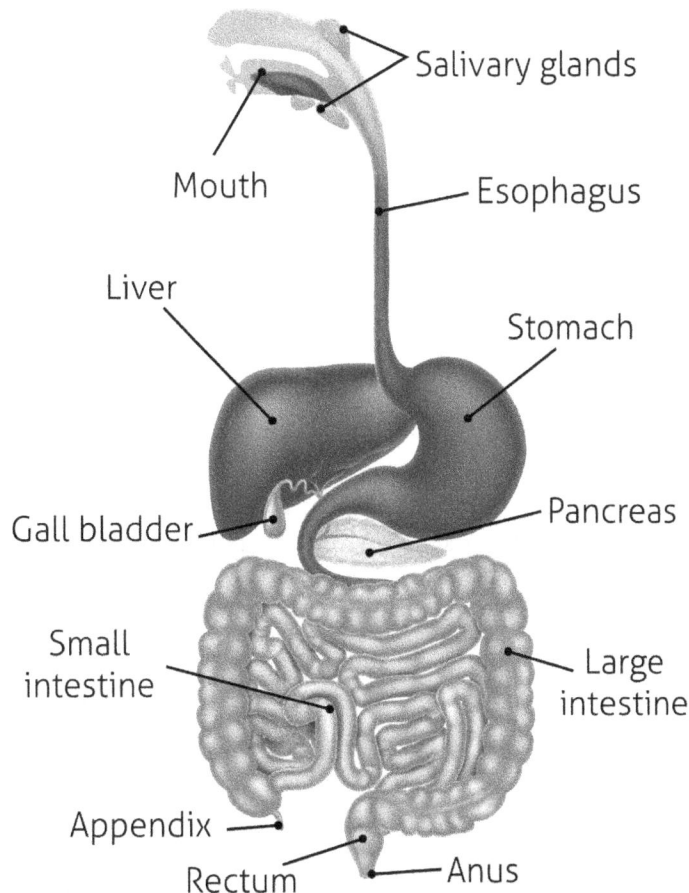

How Does Food Move Through The GI Tract?

It starts in the mouth, chewing is very important, it is the start to your food digestion. When you chew your food properly, your body releases digestive enzymes to begin the breaking down process. Your mouth is already absorbing nutrients from your food!

Then on to your tube like esophagus which pushes the contents toward the stomach. Once in the stomach the food and liquid is mixed with digestive juices, before moving the contents to the small intestine. The muscles of the small intestine mix food with digestive juices from the pancreas and liver. The small intestine pushes the mixture forward and absorbs the digested nutrients into the bloodstream, delivering the nutrients to the rest of the body.

The waste products moved to the large intestine include undigested particles of food and older cells from the GI tract. The large intestine absorbs water and any remaining nutrients and changes the waste from liquid into solid. The rectum stores it until it pushes out of the body during a hopefully successful *poo!*

[2] Endnote - *Digestive system*

So what does your digestive system have to do with your immune system? Your immune system starts in the gut. It is over 80% of your immune system and your gut flora—bacterial cells—outnumber your human cells. Gut flora lives in your digestive system but its population is very dependent on what you consume. There is a relationship between the bacteria in your body and what you feed those bacteria, based on what goes in your stomach and follows to your small intestine and large intestine. Then onto how your body uses the nutrients from all those substances coming into the digestive system.

The small intestine absorbs the nutrients from food and liquids that will be distributed by your blood stream throughout your body. We want those nutrients to be power packed with good non-inflammatory substances. Consuming inflammatory substances causes an inflammatory response that results in damage to the lining of the small intestine. Over time, this response pokes holes through that lining and it lets in food particles, toxins, and waste that would normally be too big to be absorbed.

The problems start when your body recognizes food particles that should not be in your blood stream. Some of these proteins, like gluten, are very similar to the normal proteins in the body, including those that make up our own tissue. Because these proteins are so similar, your immune system cannot distinguish between the two proteins and it begins attacking the normal tissue. This is the beginning of autoimmune disease, and the damage will keep progressing if nothing is done to address it. It is never too late to heal, repair, and even reverse some of that damage.

The FLog will help you find out what substances trigger some of your symptoms. As you eliminate those problem foods from your lifestyle, your small intestine can heal and become a more efficient barrier. Your gut flora can find harmony as you balance your diet.

Why are Some Inflammatory Foods, Well, Inflammatory?

High - Low Risk Foods

Sugar
- Causes damage leading to an extra leaky gut.
- Contributes to higher *bad* cholesterol and dreaded weight gain.
- It's addictive!

[3] Endnote - *Sugar*

Dairy
- Requires the lactase enzyme that some of us don't have, which is required to break down the sugar in milk.
- Common sensitivity to the two proteins found in milk are casein and whey.
- Many people who are gluten intolerant may also be casein intolerant.
- Ever get phlegm built up in the mouth after dairy? Yuck!

[4] Endnote - *Dairy*

Grains, Legumes, Nuts and Seeds (They are all actually seeds)
- Lectins are difficult to digest, making boiling or steaming to decrease these substances before consumption very important.
- Fermentation in the colon, creating gases. *The farts! Yikes!*
- Seeds are very high in starch because the infant plant will need a source of energy to grow.

[5] Endnote - *Grains Legumes nuts and seeds*

Alternative Sweeteners and Food Chemicals
- Artificial Sweeteners can develop into an addiction.
- Consumption of these artificial sweeteners in time can alter taste buds and dull your sense of sweet.
- Nutrient deficiencies and weight gain may increase due to the taste bud change.

[6] Endnote - *Food chemicals and additives*

Emulsifiers and Food Thickeners
- Causes inflammation because they influence certain types of bacteria to grow in your gut, this in turn disrupts the gut microbiota.
- These bacteria can be damaging to your intestine's vital mucous layer.

[7] Endnote - *Emulsifiers and food thickeners*

Nighshades
- There are chemicals in nightshade vegetables that act like a bug spray to the living plant. This is irritating to the gut lining because the chemical's sole function is to kill. It doesn't differentiate between good and bad organisms.
- In small amounts this may not cause terrible reactions, but if your lining in already damaged by other harmful foods, you're very susceptible to a leaky gut.
- If your digestive system is already compromised by an autoimmune disease you want to avoid these vegetables!

[8] Endnote - *Nightshades*

Eggs
- You may be sensitive to the proteins in egg whites, but some can't tolerate proteins in the yolk.
- Chemicals like histamines are released in the body when there is an allergic reaction, mostly from egg whites.
- Symptoms may include abdominal pain, diarrhea, or any other symptoms typical to histamine release. *Do you have skin issues? Hint, hint! Your immune system is shouting at you!*
- When chickens are fed soy and corn the chicken and its eggs become high in omega-6 fatty acids.
- You may be ok with well-cooked eggs, such as those found in baked or dry goods, but you may react negatively to *incompletely* cooked eggs. Thus when testing for sensitivities you may see a false negative.

[9] Endnote - *Eggs*

NSAID's
- Cause possible threats to your esophagus, stomach and small intestine. According to gastroenterologist Byron Cryer, MD, a spokesperson for the American Gastroenterological Association, more than half of all bleeding ulcers are caused by NSAIDs.

[10] Endnote - *NSAIDs*

Fats You Need and Fats You Don't

I couldn't have said it any better, so...here you go:

"Essential fatty acids (EFAs) are naturally occurring fats that our bodies cannot produce. Instead, they must come from whole food sources or supplements. EFAs are critical to help dampen inflammation and autoimmunity, promote blood vessel health, support healthy skin growth, give the hormones the precursors they need to remain balanced, and support healthy brain and nervous system function."

Symptoms associated with essential fatty acid deficiency:

- Poor brain function
- Painful joints; chronic pain and inflammation
- Dry, unhealthy skin and hair
- Hormone imbalances

Consume the correct ratio of Omega-6 to Omega-3 fatty acids

"It is important that your diet contains the correct ratios of different EFAs. Americans need to be most cognizant of omega-3 fatty acid, found in cold-water fish such as salmon, sardines, herring, mackerel, black cod, and bluefish. These sources contain the two most critical forms of omega-3 fatty acids, eicosapentaenoic acid (EPA) and docosahexaenoic acid (DHA)."

"DHA is vital to brain function, taming brain inflammation and preventing degeneration. Vegetarian omega-3s contain alpha-linolenic acid (ALA), which the body may convert to EPA and DHA. Dietary sources include walnuts and flax seed.

However, many people have trouble converting ALAs to beneficial forms of omega-3, particularly if insulin resistance is an issue. Eating a diet high in omega-6 fats may also hinder this conversion."

Heat can damage EFAs

"Heat is the enemy of EFAs because it changes their structure so they are less nutritious. For example, olive oil that is not heated is more nutritionally supportive than heated olive oil used for cooking. Raw fish has more usable essential fatty acids than cooked fish, and foods such as fried fish sticks offer very little in the way of essential fatty acids. Nuts that are dry-roasted or treated with heat for flavoring end up losing their essential fatty acid levels."

[11] Endnote - *Omega-3 fats*

Fats to cook with that are heat stable (Saturated Fat)
- Beef tallow or suet
- Ghee (oil separated from butter)
- Unrefined coconut oil
- Palm kernel oil...but in good conscious I can't say do this because it destroys jungles in Asia!
- Cocoa butter

Fats to heat moderately (Monounsaturated Fat)
- Bacon fat (lard)
- Butter (if you can handle the dairy)
- Duck and goose fat
- Palm Oil...but like I said...
- Chicken fat
- Olive (extra virgin) oil
- Rice bran oil

Fats to keep cool (Polyunsaturated Fat)
- Sunflower oil
- Safflower oil
- Soybean oil...*no!!*
- Corn oil (maize)...also *no.*
- Hemp oil
- Rapeseed oil (canola)
- Peanut oil...just say *no!*
- Sesame oil
- Cotton seed oil

Category Tips and Instructions

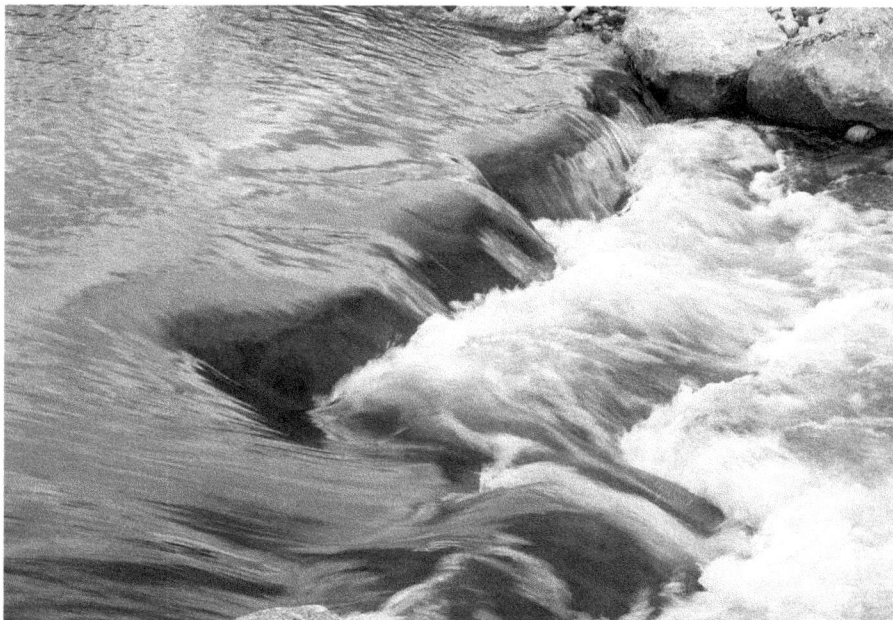

When life is rushing by and you feel you can't catch up, jump in anyway!

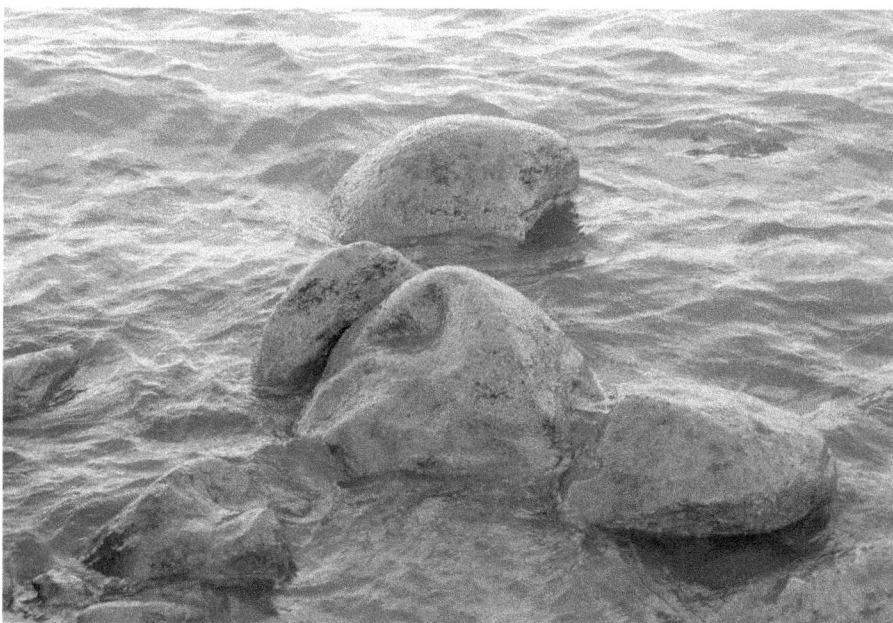

Be thankful when life is calm

Water In and Water Out

*"The Institute of Medicine sets general guidelines for total water intake. It recommends that women consume a total of 91 ounces (that's about **2.7** liters) per day—from all food and beverages combined. For men, it's about 125 ounces a day (or **3.7** liters)"*

[12] Endnote - *Water intake*

You can use tally marks to keep track of how many ounces of water you drink in a day. This excludes any other liquids, those, you list in your ingredients categories. For example, in your daily water intake section one tally mark = 8 ounces of water.

How about the fluid that comes out of your body?

Here's what your pee might be telling you:

Color
- Clear - You could actually be drinking too much water.
- Straw to clear - NORMAL.
- Dark yellow - NORMAL range but in need of more hydration.
- Honey - You need more tally marks in your daily logging - Slight dehydration.
- Brownish - Severe dehydration.
- Pink to red - Presence of blood in the urine, or possibly caused from excess consumption of vibrant colored vegetables or fruits.

Texture
- Foamy - Possible high protein in the diet could mean you are not digesting proteins well or…just go see your doctor or…maybe you just have a powerful stream from holding it too long!
- Oily - Possible excessive vitamin consumption. Pregnancy, fasting and or dehydration.

[13] Endnote - *Urine*
[14] Endnote - *Why Is My Urine Oily?*

Exercise

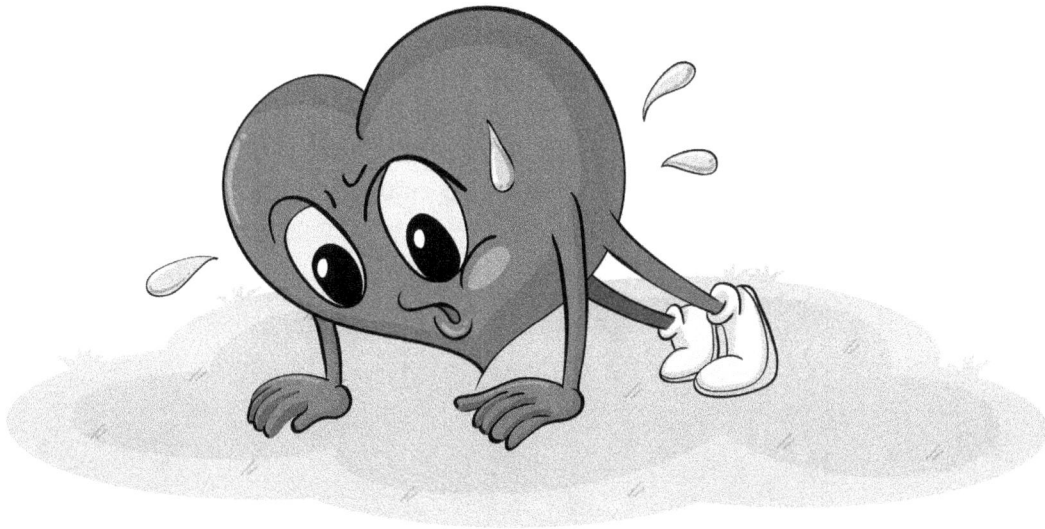

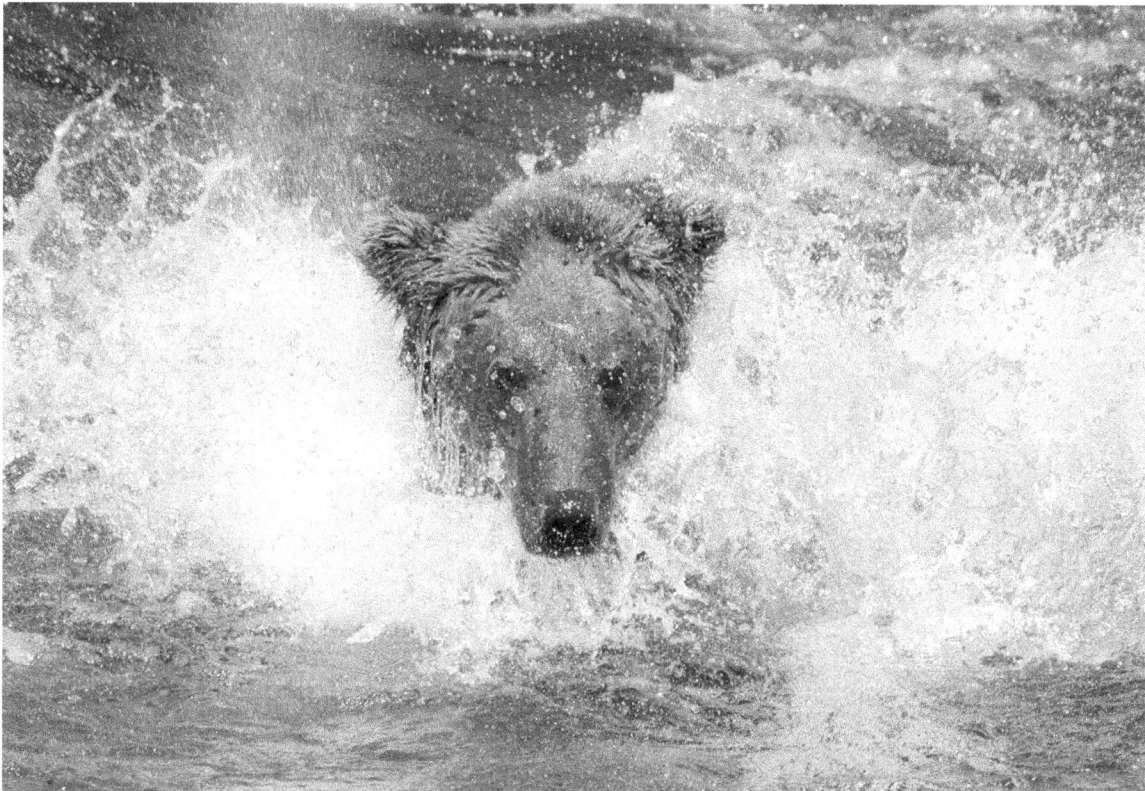

Swim even against the current

You will list the duration and what type of exercise whether:

Anaerobic: Anaerobic exercise is a physical exercise intense enough to cause lactate to form. Lactate is the conjugate base for lactic acid, used by athletes in non-endurance sports to promote strength, speed and power and by body builders to build muscle mass. Typically it would be difficult to sustain a conversation during this type of exercise.

Or

Aerobic: any of various sustained exercises, as jogging, rowing, swimming, or cycling, that stimulate and strengthen the heart and lungs, thereby improving the body's utilization of oxygen. You can still carry a conversation during this type of exercise.

Recommended durations are between 20-45 minutes and 3-5 days a week.

Strength Training and High Intensity Interval Training Over Cardio?

The answer is do what's best for you and what you enjoy most, but—*do something!* Move at a rate that will get your heart pumping faster and a little—or a lot of sweat coming out of your pores.

So whether that is yoga, a brisk walk, cross-fit games, cycling or a tough mudder—I could keep going, but you get the point. It's up to you.

FLog Your *POO!*

Stool chart

<table>
<tr><td>1.</td><td>1.</td><td>Hard, separate lumps that are difficult to pass - severe constipation.</td></tr>
<tr><td>2.</td><td>2.</td><td>Solid but lumpy, somewhat difficult to pass - mild constipation</td></tr>
<tr><td>3.</td><td>3.</td><td>Sausage like with cracks - NORMAL</td></tr>
<tr><td>4.</td><td>4.</td><td>Smooth and somewhat soft, like a hotdog - NORMAL</td></tr>
<tr><td>5.</td><td>5.</td><td>Soft blobs with clear cut edges - lacking fiber</td></tr>
<tr><td>6.</td><td>6.</td><td>Mushy consistency with ragged edges - mild diarrhea</td></tr>
<tr><td>7.</td><td>7.</td><td>Completely liquid - severe diarrhea</td></tr>
</table>

In your daily logging use the stool chart as your guide. Use the numbers to show what kind of poop experience you had and at what time of day. Your ideal numbers are 3 and 4. Don't forget to record your poop number into your symptoms category and if your experience was not up to par. What you eat or drink will affect your outcomes.

Is it a Sinker or a Floater?

It is not the weight of your stools, but rather their densities that determines their out-of-body fate to float or to sink. Simply put, the "floaters" are bloated by the air in them. Sinkers need a lot more fiber in their diet. Floaters may be caused by gas in the stool, resulting from a change in the diet. Perhaps you've suddenly started eating more high fiber foods, for example. Undigested fat will also make stools float. This could be an indication that your diet is too high in fat, or there could be a problem with nutrient absorption in your diet. Stools that result from poor food absorption often leave a greasy film on the water and are rather large. If you're suffering from constipation, you may produce impacted stools, which will "sink" because of their density and lack of moisture.

You need to include more fiber, both soluble and insoluble, in your diet to bulk out the stools and get your digestive system working properly again. And drink more water. The bowel and colon need water to work efficiently, just like the rest of your body. The truth is, a healthy stool is neither a sinker nor a floater—it's a combination of the two. If you're in good general health, you'll pass some sinkers, some floaters and some that seem to just sit in the water, neither floating nor sinking. As long as your bowel motions are soft, fairly bulky and easy and painless to pass, and there's no sign of blood or excessive mucus in the stools, everything is well down below. We want stools that do not mark the toilet bowl. We want them to hang together and not be pebbles, non-stinking, have no undigested food particles, a large volume, a clean wiping, and a definite sense of complete evacuation."

[15] Endnote - *Stool analysis*

Other Stool Concerns

Black and Tarry
- Most cases of black stools are from eating black foods or iron supplements.
- The most common condition causing black stools is a bleeding ulcer.
- Black stools caused by blood indicate a problem in the upper digestive tract.
- Black stool along with pain, vomiting, or diarrhea is cause to see a doctor right away.

[16] Endnote - *Black Tarry Stool*

Common Causes of Blood in the Stool
- Hemorrhoids
- Anal fissures

Less Common Causes of Blood in the Stool
- Colon polyps
- Inflammatory bowel disease (IBD)
- Diverticular bleeding
- Colon cancer
- Bleeding from the esophagus, stomach or small intestine

[17] Endnote - *Blood in the Stool*

Good Luck Pooping!

Stress Management

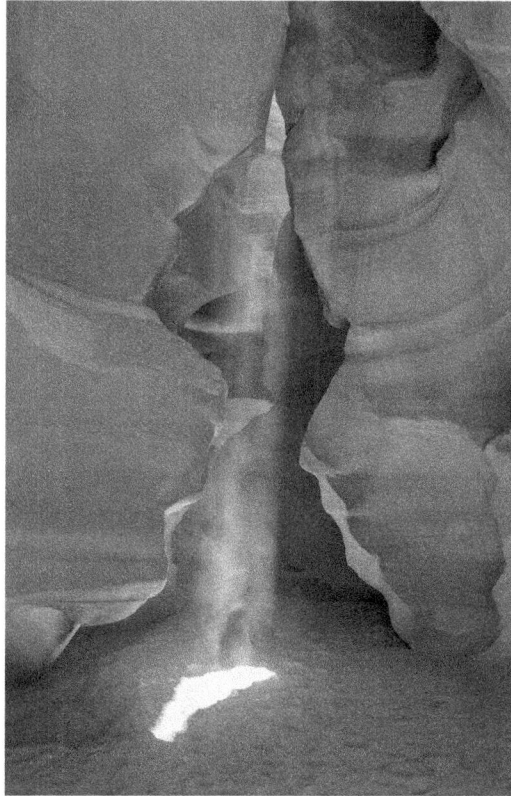

Find a ray of light in the dark…

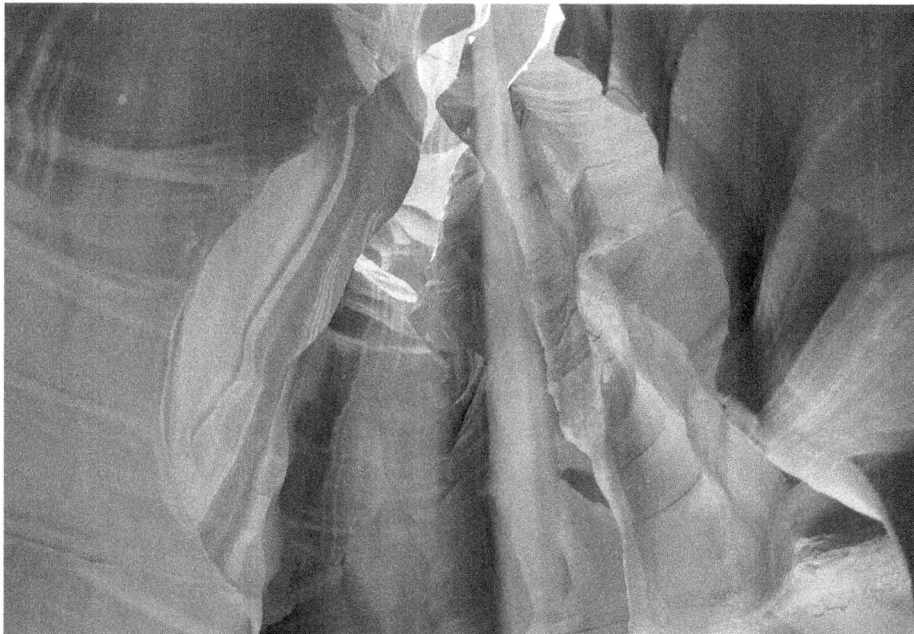

…and that light will spread

Stress comes at us in many forms. Whether it's obvious, it sneaks up on us slowly, or it's invisible. Stress indicates an imbalance between what is demanded of us and what we are able to cope with or respond to. Over time, repeated stressful situations put a strain on the body that may contribute to physical and psychological problems

Choose non-inflammatory foods, liquids and products so that:
- What you consume does not cause internal stress, which in turn causes an inflamed GI tract.
- Your body can better handle the things it can't control, including environmental stress triggers such as weather, air pollution, and bacteria that exists all around us.

External and Internal Stressors
- External stressors are in our environment like the weather, danger, hunger, isolation, the people around us or working conditions.
- Internal stressors can be from, infections, illnesses, inflammation or psychological, as in intense worry.

"The American Psychological Association conducted its most recent Stress in America Survey in 2014. A representative sample of 3,068 adults in the general population were evaluated. The survey found that overall, Americans are experiencing somewhat less stress than 7 years earlier. However, this trend is not equally shared in the population, and higher stress levels are still reported among low-income households, parents, younger generations, and women. Money appears to be the major source of high stress levels, and has impacted about one-third of Americans from leading a healthier life. Twenty percent of individuals with financial concerns are less likely to see a doctor when they need health care. They are also more likely to engage in unhealthy habits, such as lying awake at night or oversleeping, overeating, skipping meals, or becoming sedentary in general, due to stress. Emotional support was found as an important factor in helping individuals manage their stress in more effective and healthier ways."

[18] Endnote - *Stress*

Stress Hormones
- Epinephrine - Increasing your heart rate and rushes blood to your muscles and brain.
- Norepinephrine - increased blood sugar levels, also increases blood pressure but can also narrow the blood vessels, resulting in high blood pressure.

You don't want these hormones pumping all the time, creating chronic stress on the body.

[19] Endnote - *Beyond Fight or Flight*

Meditation Exercise: For 5-15 minutes: Find stillness and say thank you that you're here another day to improve your body, mind and life. You want to reach out to help others to be as well and as happy as you are. Find peace even in chaos. FLog on.

AN AUTOIMMUNE FOOD JOURNEY

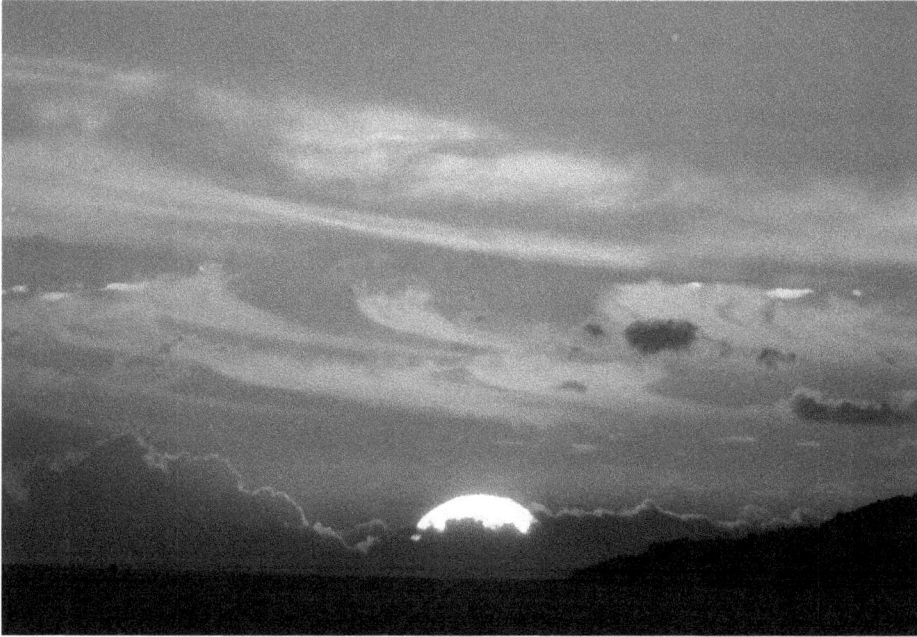

Find peace in the moment, and glory in a sunset

From The FLog's Resource Page:

Try Hypnotherapy for stress management, meditation to engage your parasympathetic nervous system, and exercise to relieve tension and help sweat out the toxins. Here are some of my favorite references for a healthy mind.
- **Surf City's hypnotherapy** applications on your electronic devices. https://surfcityapps.com
- **Meditation** with Regina Queen, http://www.intheflowwellness.com
- **Fitness Blender** on YouTube and the web for pilates, HIIT workouts, interval training for low and high impact, beginners and advanced. https://www.fitnessblender.com
- **Yoga and stretching** on YouTube for body balance and relaxation, https://www.youtube.com/watch?v=1fztE4mK7C0
- **Mobility Conditioning, MobCon**, foam roller and ball rolling with videos on YouTube for self massage, tissue release and detoxification, https://www.youtube.com/c/AngelaLPTBW

Fasting

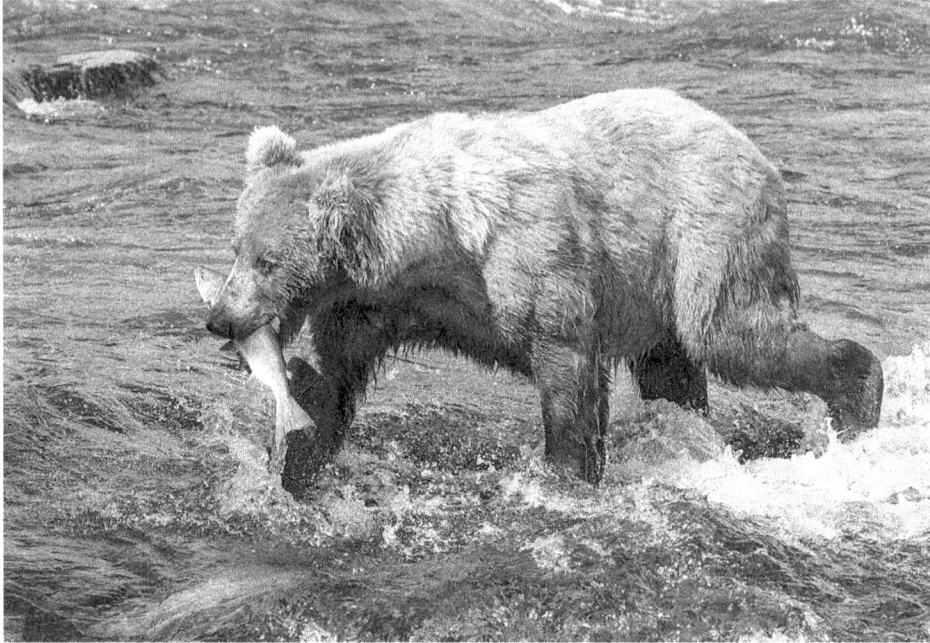

Catch 'em while you can!

The Benefits of Giving Your Body Time To Heal

The body needs quality sleep. It undergoes repair work as it sleeps. You have a repaired small intestinal lining every day you wake up from a restful sleep. By prolonging the natural fast and healing time your body takes, you promote change and you can increase fat reducing chemicals in the body. If you want to lose weight and lose belly fat, even irregular fasting could be effective.

Different Types of Fasting

Intermittent Fasting

This type of fasting is also known as cyclical fasting. Fast times range from 14 to 18 hours. Begin your fasting from 5:00pm-7:00pm the night before and have your first meal from 7:00 or 11:00 the next morning. You're sleeping through most of it!

Time-Restricted Eating

Consume no food between 12–16 hours. During your eating window, you can eat as much of your favorite healthy non-inflammatory foods as you like. This is one of the most common methods of fasting.

Time-restricted eating is pretty simple to start. If you finish dinner at 7:00pm, don't eat anything again until 7:00 or 11:00 the next morning. Again, you're sleeping through most of it.

Precautions Regarding Fasting

"The health benefits of fasting are extremely appealing, but fasting isn't always for everyone. People who suffer from hypoglycemia and diabetics should probably avoid fasting, up until blood glucose and insulin levels have been normalized. Pregnant and breastfeeding women should absolutely not fast, as it can have negative effects on the baby.

Additionally, if you are certain medications or other health conditions, it's best to consult your doctor about introducing fasting into your lifestyle. However, for most of the population, intermittent fasting can be a really helpful tool in managing your weight, body fat and gut health."

[20] Endnote - *Fasting*

Recommended Fast Protocol

Pick three separate days that work best for your schedule. Drink as much un-caffeinated non sugar based tea and water. The best herb teas to drink during fasting are peppermint, rose hips and camomile; but drinking other herb teas will be beneficial.

Drinking an organic bone broth as a supplement can help you get through the fasting period. The powerful nutrients will supply enough fuel to satisfy the low points you may experience during a day long fast. Drink as much as you need, usually 64 ounces on a 20-22 hour fast.

Bonus, you will be sleeping through half of that fasting period!

For example:
   Sunday night through Monday afternoon, 7:30pm-4:30pm fast time 20 hours
   Thursday afternoon through Friday morning, 2pm-8am fast time 18 hours
   Friday night through Saturday afternoon, 8pm-12pm fast time 16 hours

The FLog Bone Broth Recipe

Chicken Bone Broth
   1 chicken back (spine with skin and some muscle tissue attached)
   4 quarts filtered water
   1 half of an onion (whole, not chopped)
   6 celery stalks, cut in halves
   4 carrots, cut in halves
   1 green apple, cut in half
   Sea salt, small sprinkle or up to your preference
   Whole black pepper, small sprinkle or up to your preference
   1 TSP dried rosemary, parsley or oregano of your preference
   Optional apple cider vinegar, 2 tablespoons to help leech the bones

Use (preferably) an Instant Pot and set it on slow cook for the max 20 hours. Let it cool, strain, add the broth to mason jars, and store them in the refrigerator for up to a week. Usually yields 4 - 41/2 32oz jars.

If you like, take the solids of the vegetables and the apple, blending it in the blender or use a food processor. Its great for a sauce on a chicken or vegetable dish. I prefer adding some of the solids to my broth to give it texture.

Do the same for beef, pork or lamb bones and for the vegans out there, just skip the bones. Honestly, I think the veggie broth is my favorite. Add more vegetables of your choice. I prefer adding a giant chopped up yam, kale and collard greens for the vegetable broth. Discard all parts of the cooked animal carcass.

The Importance of Sleep

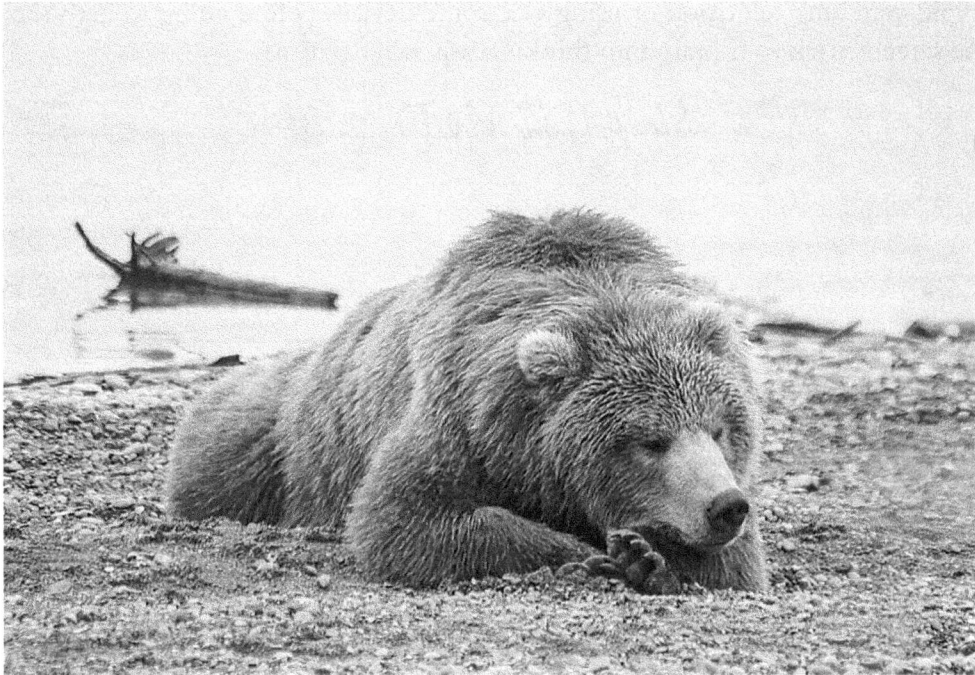

Quality sleep allows healing to occur. Make the time…

In general, most adults are designed to have sixteen hours of wakefulness and need an average of eight hours of sleep a night. The body needs adequate rest each night for a variety of reasons:
- Fighting illnesses
- Strengthening the immune system
- Repairing damaged tissues
- Digestion
- Detoxification
- Hormonal balance
- Maintaining cognitive (brain) health

Practicing the "4-7-8" breathing exercise may help. Focusing on this simple breathing method can help slow you down so you can fall asleep with ease.
- Breathe in for 4 seconds
- Hold breath for 7 seconds
- Slowly breathe out for 8 seconds

FLog Sleep Tips:
- Keep a regular sleep/wake schedule.
- Don't drink or eat caffeine four to six hours before bed and minimize daytime use.
- Don't smoke, especially close to bedtime or if you tend to wake up during the night.
- Avoid alcohol and heavy meals before sleep.
- Stretch or foam roll lightly before bed.
- Minimize noise, light, and excessive hot and cold temperatures where you sleep.

- Develop a regular bedtime and go to bed at the same time each night.
- Take 20 to 30 minutes before going to bed to relax and unwind or write down your plans for the next day. FLog, if you forgot!
- Avoid watching television or using electronic devices before going to bed: the light from the screens trick your brain into thinking it is still day time.

Sleep Well My Friends!

Shopping and Eating Tips

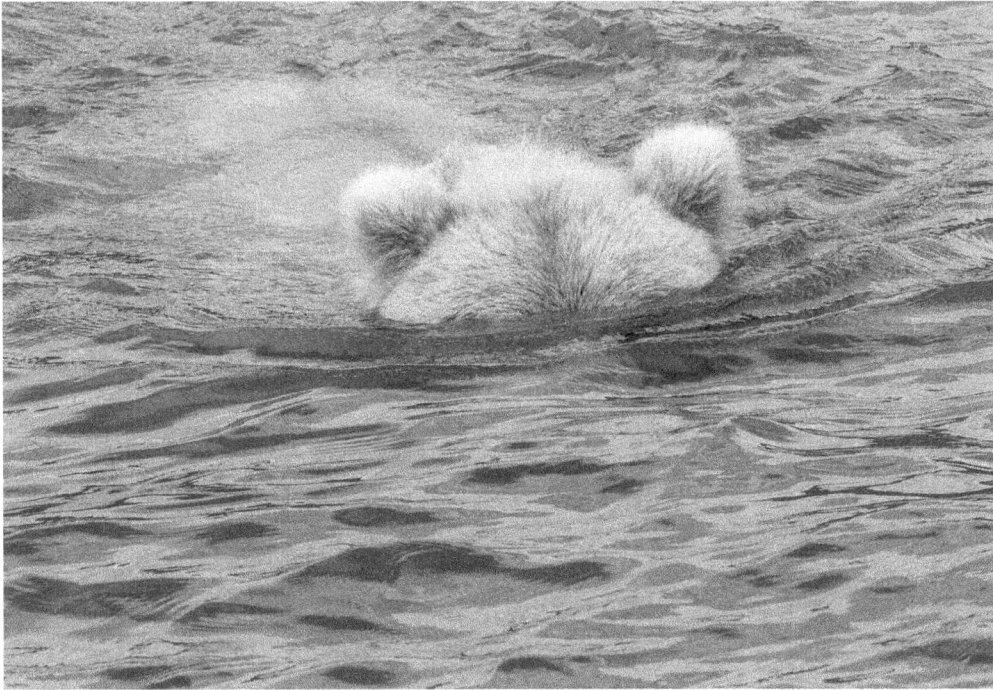

Don't get discouraged!

Going to The Market?

You've heard it a thousand times, and it's true, don't shop hungry. An empty belly often results in impulse purchases that are typically not the healthiest. Good nutrition starts long before you head to the grocery store. Plan your meals for the week and create a list to shop from. Cooking up healthy meals is a challenge if you don't have the right ingredients in your kitchen.

Most of us tend to eat the same foods over and over again. You'll notice on your grocery lists that you really tend to choose the same foods that make your body happiest. And why not? But you also need to be aware that you won't get all your nutrients if you only eat tomatoes, chicken, lettuce and that same gluten free bread all the time. For one, your choices should include a very colorful selection from the produce department. Eat your fresh green foods especially!

Here's another one you've also heard many times: shop from the outside aisles of the grocery store—the produce department, meat department, and if you're in an aisle stay with refrigerated and perishable items. Avoid the inner aisles that are full of over-processed boxes and bags of food. Frozen vegetables and fruits are preserved and still nutrient dense. If you've got big goals on your personal gut health plan, you should try to avoid eating anything that needs a label. If you do buy label food, then don't focus of what the front of the package says. Even neutral color labels make us think that the contents of the food must be healthy, because it looks 'earthy' right? Probably not, there are many ways labels may be deceiving you.

Last, try to choose organic foods whenever possible. You can refer
to your Food Law page for the dirty thirteen list.

READ THE INGREDIENTS, if you're buying label food! Make sure it's FLog legal.

Chew, Chew, Chew, That Is The Thing To Do!

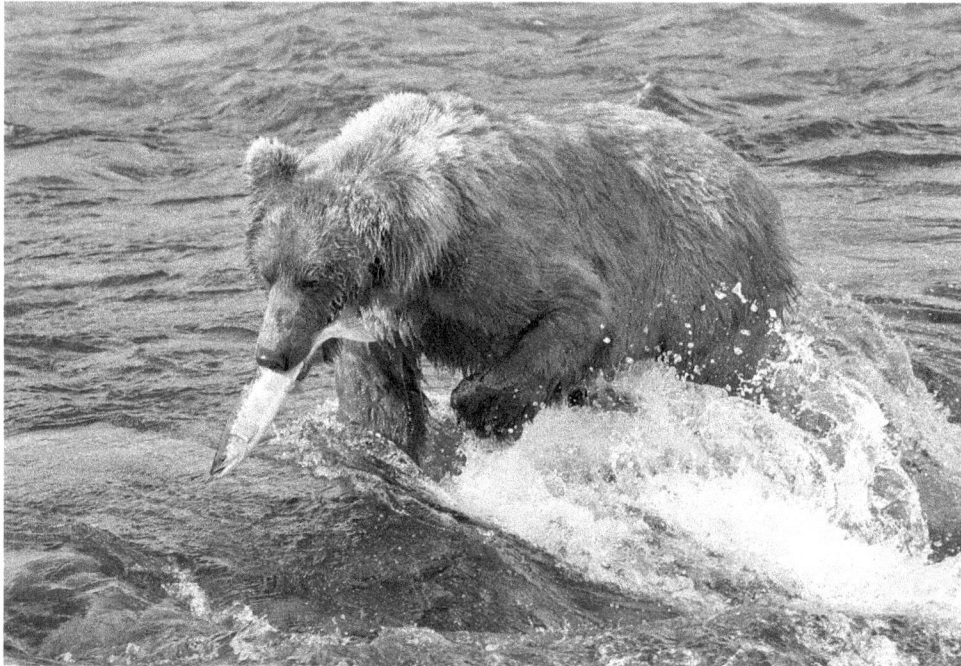

That's keeping it 100% organic

This might sound like a silly topic, but remember what your old fashioned parents (or grandparents) used to tell you when you sat at the table for a meal, "Say grace first, don't eat with your mouth open, chew your food and SLOW DOWN." They were right. You should stop and be thankful you have food to eat, and you should stop and take a look at your food choice, and decide whether you made a good decision or you "FLog failed."

Chewing your food thoroughly helps food move through the digestive tract, sending messages to the gastrointestinal system that food is on its way. This triggers hydrochloric acid production, which helps speed up the digestive process. It is also important to swallow the tiniest pieces possible. If you can still feel distinguishable parts of the food in your mouth, then keep chewing.

22 Endnote - *Chewing your food*

It takes about twenty minutes for our brain to register that we're full. If we eat fast, we can continue eating past the point where we're full. If we eat slowly, we have time to realize we're full, and stop on time. Eating slowly, and paying attention to our eating, can be a great mindfulness exercise. Be in the moment, rather than rushing through a meal thinking about what you need to do next.

Avoid distractions such as television or eating on the run so that you may be calm and focused during the meal. This also makes for a more enjoyable meal and this kind of mindfulness will help lead to a less stressful lifestyle.

Going Out to Eat

You *should* be the person at your table who asks the server all sorts of questions about the food you're paying good money for. A good server will be knowledgeable about the food served at the particular restaurant. If they don't know what types of fats the kitchen uses to cook or fry with, they should ask the cook. This will educate your server for the next person who will hopefully ask the same question. You are just participating in creating awareness, so be proud of yourself!

Many chain restaurants and some fast food locations post allergen information online or offer a separate menu. Most of the time you may need to ask for that menu. In the past few years, eating establishments have become more aware of allergies and sensitivities. I find it is best to do the research before you choose a restaurant. You can go on their website and search for their allergen list. You can also give them a call if the information is not easy to find. Feel more empowered by being prepared. Stick to restaurants that you know, which in at least my case, means less arguments over where to eat!

FOOD LAW

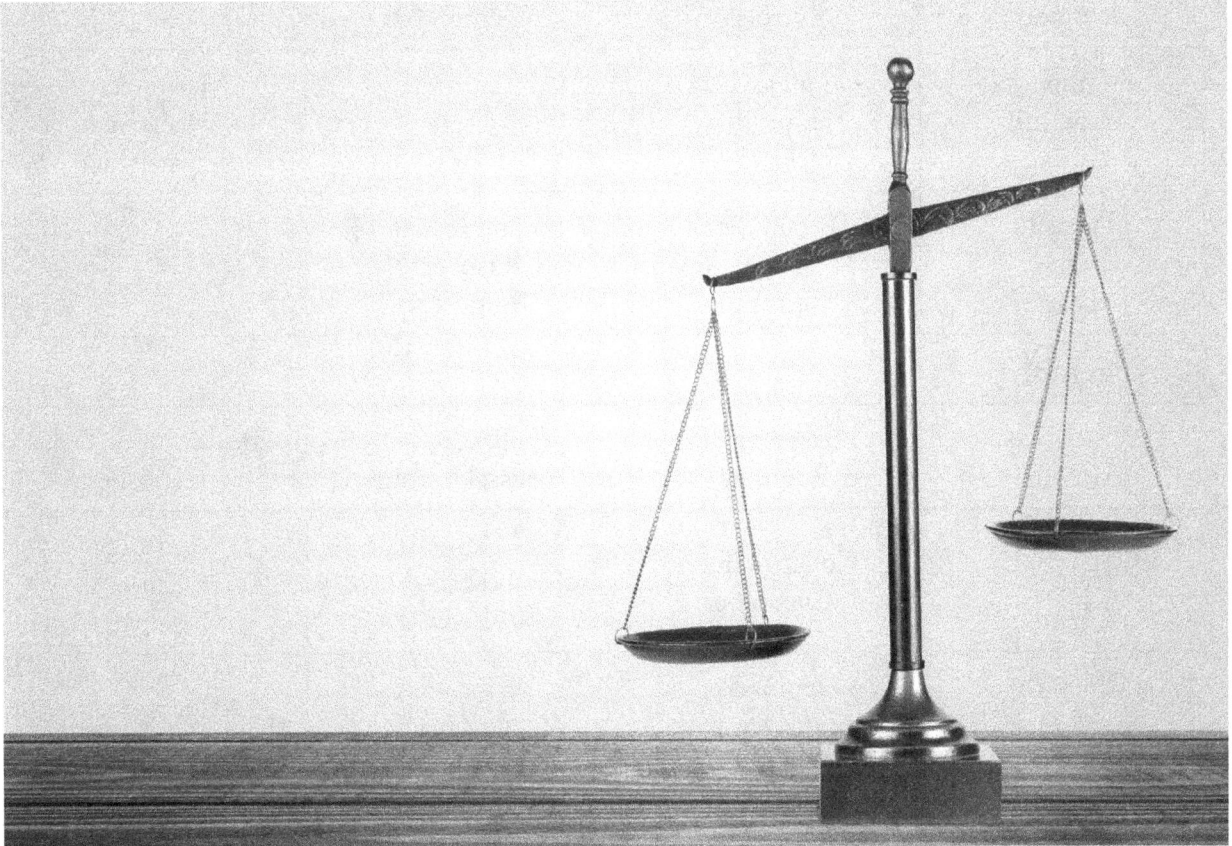

Non-Inflammatory Foods List

Foods   **To Eat**

Fruit			
Apple Apricot Avocado	Banana Blackberry Blueberry	Cantelope Cherry Clementine	Coconut Date Fig
Grape Grapefruit Guava	Honeysuckle Honeydew Kiwi	Lemon Lime Mango	Marionberry Nectarine Orange
Papaya Peach Pear	Persimmon Plum Pineapple	Pomegranate Raspberry Strawberry	Tangerine Watermelon
Vegetables			
Artichoke Arugula	Asparagus Bok Choi	Broccoli Brussel Sprouts	Butternut Squash Cabbage
Cauliflower Celery Chard	Collard Green Cucumber	Fennel Kale Leek	Lettuce Mushroom Pumpkin
Rhubarb Snap Pea	Spinach Summer Squash	Watercress Zucchini	
Roots			
Beet Carrot Jicama	Onion Parsnip Turnip	Radish Rutabaga Shallot	Sweet Potato Yam
Herbs			
Basil Bay Leaves Chives	Cilantro Lavender Lemongrass	Mint Parsley Rosemary	Sage Tarragon Thyme
Spice	**Sweeteners**		
Cinnamon Clove Ginger	Saffron Tea Turmeric	Dates Dried Organic Fruit	Maple Syrup Molassas

Other			
Apple Cider Vinegar	Anchovies Coconut Flour	Coconut Aminos	Coconut Vinegar Olives
Shirataki yam noodles	Decaf Herbal Teas: black, green, yerba mate		
Organ meat			
Bone Broth, Gizzard	Heart	Kidney	Liver
Meats*	*Always choose organic where possible	** wild caught fish, choose small ocean fish low in mercury, or fresh water fish See: (23)	
Beef Bison Buffalo	Chicken Duck Fish**	Lamb Pork Rabbit	Shellfish Turkey Venison
Fats			
Animal Fat Avocado Oil	Coconut Oil Lard	Tallow Olive Oil	
Ferments*	*Maybe ok for you/or no list if causes symptoms		
Sauerkraut Vegetables	Water Kefir	Kombucha	

[23] *Mercury and fish*

Pro-Inflammatory Foods List

Foods	To Avoid		
All grains			
Barley Bulgur	Wheat Corn	Durum Wheat	Millet Oats Popcorn
Kamut Rice	Rye Einkorn	Emmer Farro Fonio	Sorghum Spelt
Teff Triticale	Wheat Wild Rice		
Dairy			
Butter Buttermilk	Cheese Condensed Milk	Cream Cream Cheese	Yogurt Goat Cheese
Legumes	Beans, including peanuts		
Abzuki Beans	Black Beans	Black-eyed Peas	Broad Beans
Chick Peas	Fava Beans	Garbanzo Beans	Kidney Beans
Lima Beans	Mung Beans	Navy Beans	Peanuts
Soy Beans/Tofu	White Beans		
Alternative Sweeteners	**Sugar**, other than allowed fruits		
Aspartame Equal Lactitol	Erythritol Glycyrrhizin	Glycerol Maltitol	Mannitol Neotame
NutraSweet Polydextrose	Saccharin Somalt	Sorbitol Splenda	Sucralose Truvia
Tagatose	Xylitol		

"Maybe OK for You" Foods

If you are going to choose food from the low risk list, then you should only be choosing organic forms free of mold. Pick a reputable company with excellent processing procedures and strict cross contamination regulations. Nuts and seeds should be raw and not roasted (cooked) in order to properly soak or sprout.

Nuts	See soaking and sprouting list		
Almond Brazil Cashew	Hazelnut Pecan Cocoa	Pine Nut Pistachio	Macadamia Walnut
Seeds	See soaking and sprouting list		
Anise Canola Caraway	Chia Coriander Cumin	Fennel Fenugreek Flax	Mustard Nutmeg Poppy
Pumpkin Sesame	Sunflower Hemp	Coffee (bean)	
Eggs (white or yolk)			
Chicken	Duck	Goose	Quail
Other			
Alcohol	Stevia	Thickeners	Sugar
Malt Vinegar	Green beans Snow peas	Whole bean organic coffee	Coconut milk or water
Nightshades			
Cayenne Pepper Chili Pepper	Chili Chipotle	Eggplant Goji Berry	Ground Cherry Habanero Pepper
Jalepeno Pepper Paprika	Poblano Pepper Potato	Sweet Pepper Tobacco	Tamatillo Tomato
Wolf Berry			

Do your best to choose all organic foods, especially: all animal protein and fats. When shopping for produce use the below guides.

Clean 15	Little need for pesticides		
Avocados Asperagus	Cabbage Cantelope Eggplant	Grapefruit Kiwi Mango	Onion Pineapple Sweet Corn
Sweet Onion	Sweet Potato	Sweet Peas	Watermelon

Dirty 13	Contains the most pesticides		
Apples Cherries	Celery Collard Greens	Domestic Blueberries Imported Grapes	Kale Lettuce
Nectarines Peaches	Potato Sweet Bell Peppers	Spinach	

If you decide these ingredients do not cause symptoms, nuts, seeds or grains should be in raw form and freshly soaked or sprouted to remove or reduce their naturally protective barrier, called phytic acid.

SOAKING AND SPROUTING			
Soak	Time	Sprout	Time
Almonds	8hrs	NO	None
Barley	6hrs	YES	2 days
Buckwheat	6hrs	YES	2 days
Chickpeas	8hrs	YES	2-3 days
Flax Seeds	1/2hr	NO	None
Kamut	7hrs	YES	2-3 days
Lentil Beans	7hrs	YES	3 days

SOAKING AND SPROUTING			
Oat Groats	6hrs	YES	2 days
Quinoa	2hrs	YES	1 day
Rye	8hrs	YES	3 days
Sesame Seeds	6hrs	YES	2 days
Spelt	7hrs	YES	2 days
Walnuts	4hrs	NO	None
Wheat Berries	7hrs	YES	2-3 days
Wild Rice	9hrs	YES	3-5 days
All other nuts	6hrs	NO	None

RISK LIST (Cut out of book)

Post in your kitchen, at work or any where it would help to be reminded.

HIGH RISK			
All grains			
Barley Bulgur	Wheat Corn	Durum Wheat	Millet Oats
Popcorn Kamut	Rice Rye	Einkorn Emmer	Farro Fonio
Semolina Wheat	Sorghum Spelt	Teff Triticale	Wheat Wild Rice
Dairy			
Butter Buttermilk	Cheese Condensed Milk	Cream Cream Cheese	Yogurt Goat Cheese
Legumes	Beans, including peanuts		
Abzuki Beans	Black Beans	Black-eyed Peas	Broad Beans
Chick Peas	Fava Beans	Garbanzo Beans	Kidney Beans
Lima Beans	Mung Beans	Navy Beans	Peanuts
Soy Beans/Tofu	White Beans		
Alternative Sweeteners	**Sugar**, other than allowed fruits		
Aspartame Equal	Erythritol Lactitol	Glycyrrhizin Glycerol	Maltitol Mannitol
Neotame NutraSweet	Polydextrose Saccharin	Somalt Sorbitol	Splenda Sucralose
Truvia Tagatose	Xylitol		

MEDIUM RISK			
NSAID's			
Aspirin	Ibuprofen	Naproxen	
Emulsifiers/ thickeners			
Agar Albumin Alginates	Casein Ceatyl Alcohol	Cholic acid Cellulose Gum	Desoxycholic acid
Egg Yolk Lecithin	Diacetyl tartaric acid esters	Guar Gum Glycerol Gums	Irish Moss (carrageenan)
Mono - and diglycerides	Monosodium phosphate	Monostearate	Ox bile extract
Propylene glycol Soaps	Soy Lecithin	Taurocholic acid or its sodium salt	Zanthan Gum
Food Chemicals			
1-Methylcyclopropene	Artificial Colors	Aspartame	Astaxanthin
Benzoic Acid/ Sodium Benzoate	BHA - Butylated Hydroxyanisole/ toluene	Canthaxanthin	Emulsifiers
High Fructose Corn Syrup	MSG, Monosodium Glutamate	Partially Hydrogenated Oils	Potassium Bromate
Sodium Nitrate and Nitrate			
"Natural flavors" or "spices"	Beware of dressings, sauces and condiments	Avoid: Chewing gum, bouillon, brewer's yeast	

[24] Endnote - *Food chemicals and additives*
[25] Endnote - *NSAIDs*

LOW RISK			
All eggs*	*These are also in the Maybe OK for you list		
Chicken	Duck	Goose	Quail
Nuts and seeds*, see soaking and sprouting list	*These are also in the maybe ok for you list		
Almond Brazil Cashew	Cocoa Hazelnut Pecan	Pine Nut Pistachio	Macadamia Walnut
Anise Canola Caraway	Chia Coriander Cumin	Fennel Fenugreek Flax	Mustard Nutmeg
Poppy Pumpkin	Sesame Sunflower	Hemp	Coffee (bean)
Other			
Alcohol	Coconut milk or water	Ghee	Green beans Snow peas
Malt Vinegar	Whole bean organic coffee	Thickeners	
Nightshades*	*These maybe ok for you, but are by nature inflammatory		
Capsicum Cayenne pepper	Eggplant Goji berries	Gooseberries Ground Cherries	Okra Paprika
Peppers Pepino melons	Sorrel Tobacco	Tomatillo Tomatoes	
Wolf Berry			

FODMAPs

You only need to score foods on the FODMAP's list if:
- They are also in any of the risk categories
- If they actually cause symptoms or if you suspect they may cause symptoms. Remember to list all foods you react to or suspect you reacted to on your 'Noticing a Pattern?' log pages.

What are FODMAP's?

First of all most people don't need to follow this list unless they have SIBO (small intestinal bacterial overgrowth, yeast overgrowth or IBS (irritable bowel syndrome) but if you're FLogging then you're watching out for reactions to all foods. Hopefully this list helps you figure it out! Only score these foods once you start seeing a pattern of symptoms.

FODMAPs *"are a collection of short chain carbohydrates and sugar alcohols found in foods naturally or as food additives. FODMAPs include fructose (when in excess of glucose), fructans, galacto-oligosaccharides (GOS), lactose and polyols (eg. sorbitol and mannitol). A detailed description of each of these, including the foods they are found in, is provided below.*

A diet low in FODMAPs ("a Low FODMAP Diet") is scientifically, and is now used internationally, as the most effective dietary therapy for Irritable Bowel Syndrome (IBS) and symptoms of an irritable bowel. Such symptoms include excessive wind (flatus), abdominal pain, bloating and distention, nausea and changes in bowel habits (diarrhea and/or constipation). A Low FODMAP Diet has also been proven, with solid scientific evidence, to reduce symptoms of fatigue, lethargy and poor concentration."

FODMAP is an acronym that stands for:
Fermentable – meaning they are broken down (fermented) by bacteria in the large bowel
Oligosaccharides – "oligo" means "few" and "saccharide" means sugar. These molecules made up of individual sugars joined together in a chain
Disaccharides – "di" means two. This is a double sugar molecule.
Monosaccharides – "mono" means single. This is a single-sugar molecule.
And
Polyols – these are sugar alcohols

FODMAPs			
Legumes			
Abzuki Beans	Black Beans	Black-eyed Peas	Broad Beans
Chick Peas	Fava Beans	Garbanzo Beans	Kidney Beans

FODMAPs			
Lima Beans	Mung Beans	Navy Beans	Peanuts
Soy Beans/Tofu	White Beans		
Fruits			
Apples Apricot Avocado	Blackberries Figs Goji	Grapefruit Guava Lychee	Mango Peaches
Persimmon Plums Pomegranate	Prunes Raisins	Sultanes Tamarillo	Watermelon
Dairy			
Kefir and sheep's milk			
Vegetables			
Artichoke Asparagus	Beetroot Cassava	Cauliflower Celery	Garlic Mushrooms
Onions (white parts)	Peas Shallots		
Grains and nuts			
Amaranth Barley Carob	Granola Gnocchi Oats	Muesli Rye	Spelt Sourdough
Meats			
Deli	Chorizo	Processed meats	Sausages (cured meats)
Sweeteners			
Agave High fructose corn syrup Honey	Inulin Isomalt	Maltitol Mannitol	Sorbitol Xylitol
Prebiotics			

FODMAPs			
Inulin Oligofructose	Fructooligosaccharides		
Drinks			
Beer Coconut Water Chia	Cordial-apple raspberry or orange	Fruit juices Teas with apple	Rum Sodas
Black tea Dandelion Fennel	Chamomile Herbal Oolong tea	Wine Whey	
Other			
Tahini	Pesto	Tzatziki	

[26] Endnote - *Fodmaps*

For example:

High FODMAP containing foods

Excess fructose

Fruits: Apples, cherries, mango, pears, tinned fruit in natural fruit juice, watermelon, large quantities of fruit juice or dried fruit

Vegetables: Asparagus, artichokes, sugar snap peas

Sugars: Honey, high fructose corn syrup

Lactose

Milk & Yogurts: Regular and low fat milk and yogurts

Dairy Products: Soft cheeses (e.g. ricotta, cottage, cream cheese); custard, ice-cream

Fructans (fructo-oligosaccharides) & Galacto-oligosaccharides

Grains: Rye and rye products (e.g. rye bread, rye crackers); Wheat and wheat products (wheat bread, pasta, couscous, wheat bran)

Fruits: Peaches, persimmon, watermelon

Vegetables: Artichokes, legumes (baked beans, lentils, red kidney beans); onion and garlic and garlic salts

Others: Inulin (often called fiber in nutritional supplements and products)

Polyols – Sorbitol

Fruits: Apples, apricots, pears, blackberries, nectarines, plums

Beverages: Apple and pear juice

AN AUTOIMMUNE FOOD JOURNEY

Polyols – Mannitol
> Vegetables: Cauliflower, mushrooms, snow peas
> Fruits: Watermelon

Polyols – Sorbitol & Mannitol
> Sweeteners: Sugar-free gums, hard candies and chocolates containing sorbitol, mannitol, xylitol isomalt, maltitol

[27] Endnote - *Measuring FODMAPs*

The reason processed meats are listed is because processed meats usually contain extra ingredients, such as seasonings, garlic and onion, etc.

Keeping Score

Your FLog score will help you connect the dots between certain foods and symptoms. You can then reduce these foods from your diet or completely remove them based on the frequency or severity of the symptoms. The idea is to remove inflammatory food from your diet so your digestive system can heal, resulting in an immune system ready to face the world's harsh environment. Even if you do not feel obvious symptoms from any of the risk food groups, continue to grade yourself to keep track of the quantity of inflammatory substances you consume on a regular basis. Some delayed reactions simply are quantitative in nature: the more junk you pile on, the harder your system needs to work to detoxify.

Use the 'Favorite Unique Food Routine' log pages to record what you eat often and all its ingredients. Ideally, the foods you consume should contain the least amount of points.

You should take the FLog with you during your day so you can log on the go and at work. However if carrying an extra item with you is impractical, you can take pictures of your food or drinks and log them later. If you had a meal, snack or drink that had a label of ingredients, then you should snap a photo of that label to record later. If you post your food pictures on social media don't forget to use the hashtag #theflogjourney.

FLog Instructions:
1. Keep a record of what you eat and drink throughout the day.
2. Add a point for each inflammatory ingredient on the 'Risk Food' lists (see Food Law pages).
3. You will then add up the total number of inflammatory substances you consumed during that window of time. For example:

Time	4am-11am
FOOD Solid	List ingredients, be descriptive but don't overthink it.
or liquid	Take a photo of the list of ingredients if needed. (If you ate label food)
Score: 5	Eggs, spinach, mushroom, coconut butter for cooking, gluten free bagel-4 (Teff, maltodextrin, sorghum, corn syrup) strawberry jam and coconut butter Peanut butter-1 celery, banana

At the end of the day add together all four scores to create your day's grade.

A+	A	A-	B+	B	B-
0	1-2	3-4	5-6	7-9	10-12
C+	C	C-	D+	D	F
13-15	16-18	19-21	22-24	25-27	28+

Your FLog Report Card

A+ is your ultimate goal, but can you do it everyday? Human nature says its not likely, so challenge yourself to do it:

    1-2 days a week
    3 days in a row
    5 days in a row

A, - A- You're getting control!
Challenge yourself to do it:

    1- 2 days a week
    3 days in a row
    5 days in a row
    7 days in a row

B+ - C+ Almost there!
Challenge yourself to do it:

    3 days in a row
    5 days in a week

C, - C+ You've got to do better!
Challenge yourself to do it:

    1 day a week
    3 days in a week

D+ - D Baby stepper!
    Challenge yourself to do it:
    1 day a week or less

F Your immune system is in the "Danger Zone" if you do this too many days in a row. WTFLog are you thinking?
Challenge yourself to do it:

    2 days or 0 in a month!

Within three to six weeks, you should have a detailed list of foods and reactions on your 'Noticing A Pattern' pages. Add a point to your daily grade even if you can eat certain 'Risk Foods' without reactions. Remember, the immune system can change and those foods may affect you at some point because of their inflammatory nature. Always count a point to your daily score for *any* 'Risk foods.'

- If you have an autoimmune condition, disease or infection of any kind or even cancer I strongly urge you to eliminate 'Risk foods' from your diet to keep inflammation and your immune system under control.
- If you don't have a diagnosis but suffer mild symptoms from any category on the reactions and symptoms list, I suggest you adhere to the 'Maybe Ok For You' list and follow its instructions. Consider them a 'Risk Food' if you notice a pattern of symptoms after eating these foods.
- If you are trying the FLog simply for your well being, I congratulate you on seeking better health. I suggest the same for you as I did in the above category. You're fortunate to have a super hero immune system and metabolism. Choose organic, whole foods as your preventative food medicine.

Symptoms and Reactions List

Fill in any symptoms or reactions you may have if not listed

Digestive			
Diarrhea Constipation Nausea Gas	Heartburn Bloating Cramps Indigestion	Burping Phlegm Acid Reflux	GERD Intense cravings Weight gain/ Belly fat
Fill in:	Fill in:	Fill in:	Fill in:
Fill in:	Fill in:	Fill in:	Fill in:

Cognitive/ Cerebral			
Anxiety Headache Sleeplessness	Brain fog Depression	ADD/ADHD Anger	Lack of focus Vertigo
Fatigue Hearling Loss	Memory loss Vision Loss	Vision blurred, spots	Fill in:
Fill in:	Fill in:	Fill in:	Fill in:
Fill in:	Fill in:	Fill in:	Fill in:

Body			
Acne Swelling Congested	Hives Muscle Pain Nose Run	Rash: Psoriasis Rosacea or Eczema	Numbness or tingling

Body			
Nose Bleed Sweating Joint Pain	Itching (genital, rectal, skin)	Excessive body odor, or bad breath	Dry eye or mouth
Infections	Illness:	Allergies	Sleep Paralysis
Hair Loss Back Pain	High blood Pressure	Gout	Arthritis
Nail Fungus	Gingivitis Oral health issues	Athlete's Foot	Fill in:
Fill in:	Fill in:	Fill in:	Fill in:

Record Keeping
Noticing a Pattern?

Fill in your most common foods that produce a symptom and how often you have been affected. This is pretty specific, so at this point you have figured out which ingredient or product it is.

Notice your pattern after three entries? It's time to keep this ingredient on the _no_ list of foods. You can give it a try once in a while but make sure you record any reaction, then make the final wise decision to permanently strike it from your life. Consider any topical products such as skin care, hair care, make up, air fresheners, etc that also contain these ingredients. You may not want to ever use them. You can list those products here as well if it creates a symptom/reaction.

Gluten

Date/reaction: _____

Date reaction: _____

Date/reaction: _____

Date/reaction: _____

Soy

Date/reaction:_____

Date reaction: _____

Date/reaction: _____

Date/reaction: _____

Corn

Date/reaction: _____

Date reaction: _____

Date/reaction: _____

Date/reaction: _____

Dairy

Date/reaction: _____

Date reaction: _____

Date/reaction: _____

Date/reaction: _____

Ingredient and/or product brand: _____

Date/reaction: _____

Date reaction: _____

Date/reaction: _____

Date/reaction: _____

Ingredient and/or product brand: _____

Date/reaction: _____

Date reaction: _____

Date/reaction: _____

Date/reaction: _____

Ingredient and/or product brand: _____

Date/reaction: _____

Date reaction: _____

Date/reaction: _____

Date/reaction: _____

Ingredient and/or product brand: _____

Date/reaction: _____

Date reaction: _____

Date/reaction: _____

Date/reaction: _____

Ingredient and/or product brand: _____

Date/reaction: _____

Date reaction: _____

Date/reaction: _____

Date/reaction: _____

Ingredient and/or product brand: _____

Date/reaction: _____

Date reaction: _____

Date/reaction: _____

Date/reaction: _____

Ingredient and/or product brand: _____

Date/reaction: _____

Date reaction: _____

Date/reaction: _____

Date/reaction: _____

Ingredient and/or product brand: _____

Date/reaction: _____

Date reaction: _____

Date/reaction: _____

Date/reaction: _____

Ingredient and/or product brand: _____

Date/reaction: _____

Date reaction: _____

Date/reaction: _____

Date/reaction: _____

Ingredient and/or product brand: _____

Date/reaction: _____

Date reaction: _____

Date/reaction: _____

Date/reaction: _____

Ingredient and/or product brand: _____

Date/reaction: _____

Date reaction: _____

Date/reaction: _____

Date/reaction: _____

Ingredient and/or product brand: _____

Date/reaction: _____

Date reaction: _____

Date/reaction: _____

Date/reaction: _____

Ingredient and/or product brand: _____

Date/reaction: _____

Date reaction: _____

Date/reaction: _____

Date/reaction: _____

Ingredient and/or product brand: _____

Date/reaction: _____

Date reaction: _____

Date/reaction: _____

Date/reaction: _____

Ingredient and/or product brand: _____

Date/reaction: _____

Date reaction: _____

Date/reaction: _____

Date/reaction: _____

Ingredient and/or product brand: _____

Date/reaction: _____

Date reaction: _____

Date/reaction: _____

Date/reaction: _____

Ingredient and/or product brand: _____

Date/reaction: _____

Date reaction: _____

Date/reaction: _____

Date/reaction: _____

Ingredient and/or product brand: _____

Date/reaction: _____

Date reaction: _____

Date/reaction: _____

Date/reaction: _____

Ingredient and/or product brand: _____

Date/reaction: _____

Date reaction: _____

Date/reaction: _____

Date/reaction: _____

Ingredient and/or product brand: _____

Date/reaction: _____

Date reaction: _____

Date/reaction: _____

Date/reaction: _____

Ingredient and/or product brand: _____

Date/reaction: _____

Date reaction: _____

Date/reaction: _____

Date/reaction: _____

Ingredient and/or product brand: _____

Date/reaction: _____

Date reaction: _____

Date/reaction: _____

Date/reaction: _____

Ingredient and/or product brand: _____

Date/reaction: _____

Date reaction: _____

Date/reaction: _____

Date/reaction: _____

Ingredient and/or product brand: _____

Date/reaction: _____

Date reaction: _____

Date/reaction: _____

Date/reaction: _____

Ingredient and/or product brand: _____
Date/reaction: _____
Date reaction: _____
Date/reaction: _____
Date/reaction: _____

Ingredient and/or product brand: _____
Date/reaction: _____
Date reaction: _____
Date/reaction: _____
Date/reaction: _____

Ingredient and/or product brand: _____
Date/reaction: _____
Date reaction: _____
Date/reaction: _____
Date/reaction: _____

Ingredient and/or product brand: _____
Date/reaction: _____
Date reaction: _____
Date/reaction: _____
Date/reaction: _____

Ingredient and/or product brand: _____
Date/reaction: _____
Date reaction: _____
Date/reaction: _____
Date/reaction: _____

Ingredient and/or product brand: _____
Date/reaction: _____
Date reaction: _____
Date/reaction: _____
Date/reaction: _____

Favorite Unique Food Routines

These pages are for you to list your favorite food recipes, or just foods you eat often. Give it a nickname or name the brand and you won't have to re-list the ingredients every time you eat them. Hopefully you're creating only good habits and you will not need to calculate any bad scores from this list! Be disciplined.

If you have found your favorite recipes, keep that record on these pages. Write down the page number and book you found it in, or the website you found it on. List all the ingredients even if it comes from label food. It better be clean and non-inflammatory!

What's it called: _____

Ingredients: _____

_____

_____

_____

Book, page number or website: _____

What's it called: _____

Ingredients: _____

_____

_____

_____

Book, page number or website: _____

What's it called: _____

_____

_____

_____

Book, page number or website: _____

What's it called: _____

_____

_____

_____

Book, page number or website: _____

What's it called: _____

_____

_____

_____

Book, page number or website: _____

What's it called: _____

_____

_____

_____

Book, page number or website:

What's it called: _____

_____

_____

_____

Book, page number or website: _____

What's it called: _____

_____

_____

_____

Book, page number or website:_____

What's it called:

_____

_____

_____

Book, page number or website: _____

What's it called: _____

_____

_____

_____

Book, page number or website: _____

What's it called:_____

_____

_____

_____

Book, page number or website: _____

What's it called: _____

_____

_____

_____

Book, page number or website: _____

What's it called: _____

_____

_____

_____

Book, page number or website: _____

What's it called: _____

_____

_____

_____

Book, page number or website: _____

What's it called:

_____

_____

Book, page number or website: _____

What's it called: _____

_____

_____

_____

Book, page number or website: _____

What's it called: _____

_____

_____

_____

Book, page number or website: _____

What's it called: _____

_____

_____

_____

Book, page number or website: _____

Supplements and/or Medication

List each of what you take each day, when you started it, your regularity of use and what you hope to achieve by taking it.

As your health improves through your change in diet and lifestyle consider whether you still need to be taking them as often, at the same dose or ever. Consult your healthcare provider on all supplements and before considering changes to your medication. Do some research on any ingredients in your supplements or medication that you may be sensitive or reactive to.

Be your own advocate for your health!

Supplement or medication, include dosage: _____

Date you started: _____

Date you ended or any changes: _____

Regularity of when you take it: _____

Why it should be beneficial and what you hope to achieve: _____

_____

_____

_____

Supplement or medication, include dosage: _____

Date you started: _____

Date you ended or any changes: _____

Regularity of when you take it: _____

Why it should be beneficial and what you hope to achieve: _____

_____

_____

_____

Supplement or medication, include dosage: _____

Date you started: _____

Date you ended or any changes: _____

Regularity of when you take it: _____

Why it should be beneficial and what you hope to achieve: _____

_____

_____

_____

Supplement or medication: _____

Date you started: _____

Date you ended or any changes: _____

Regularity of when you take it: _____

Why it should be beneficial and what you hope to achieve: _____

_____

_____

_____

Supplement or medication: _____

Date you started: _____

Date you ended or any changes: _____

Regularity of when you take it: _____

Why it should be beneficial and what you hope to achieve: _____

_____

_____

_____

Supplement or medication: _____

Date you started: _____

Date you ended or any changes: _____

Regularity of when you take it: _____

Why it should be beneficial and what you hope to achieve: _____

_____

_____

_____

Supplement or medication: _____

Date you started:_____

Date you ended or any changes:_____

Regularity of when you take it: _____

Why it should be beneficial and what you hope to achieve: _____

_____

_____

_____

Supplement or medication:_____

Date you started:_____

Date you ended or any changes:_____

Regularity of when you take it:_____

Why it should be beneficial and what you hope to achieve: _____

_____

_____

_____

Supplement or medication:_____

Date you started:_____

Date you ended or any changes:_____

Regularity of when you take it: _____

Why it should be beneficial and what you hope to achieve: _____

_____

_____

_____

Supplement or medication:_____

Date you started: _____

Date you ended or any changes:_____

Regularity of when you take it:_____

Why it should be beneficial and what you hope to achieve: _____

_____

_____

_____

Supplement or medication: _____

Date you started: _____

Date you ended or any changes: _____

Regularity of when you take it: _____

Why it should be beneficial and what you hope to achieve: _____

_____

_____

_____

Supplement or medication:_____

Date you started:_____

Date you ended or any changes: _____

Regularity of when you take it: _____

Why it should be beneficial and what you hope to achieve: _____

_____

_____

_____

Supplement or medication:_____

Date you started: _____

Date you ended or any changes: _____

Regularity of when you take it: _____

Why it should be beneficial and what you hope to achieve: _____

_____

_____

_____

Supplement or medication, include dosage:_____

Date you started:_____

Date you ended or any changes:_____

Regularity of when you take it: _____

Why it should be beneficial and what you hope to achieve: _____

_____

_____

_____

Supplement or medication, include dosage: _____

Date you started: _____

Date you ended or any changes: _____

Regularity of when you take it:_____

Why it should be beneficial and what you hope to achieve: _____

_____

_____

_____

Your	A year for change A month for change A week for change A day for change Day 1	FLog

Date:	*Viva La FLog!*	M T W TH F Sa Su

Sleep	Hours, time, quality, dreams, any A.M. symptoms? Circle a face: ☺ ☺ 😐 ☹ 😖

Time to eat: Solid or liquid Score:	4am - 11am, List all ingredients, be descriptive but don't over think it.

Symptoms:	How do you feel? See symptoms chart.

Time to eat: Solid or liquid Score:	11am - 4pm, List all ingredients

Symptoms:	How do you feel? See symptoms chart.

Time to eat: Solid or liquid Score:	4pm - 8pm, List all ingredients

Symptoms:	How do you feel? See symptoms chart.
Time to eat: **Solid or** **liquid** **Score:**	8pm - 4am, List all ingredients
Symptoms:	How do you feel? See symptoms chart.

H2O Per 8oz	Exercise, Minutes and type Anaerobic:	Minutes and type Aerobic:	Stool Analysis, time, type and the face you made
Supplements and/ or medication, other medical related logging AM: YES/NO PM: YES/NO			☺ ☺ ☺ ☹ 😖 ☺ ☺ ☺ ☹ 😖 ☺ ☺ ☺ ☹ 😖
Notes, thoughts and goals for the day ☺ ☺ ☺ ☹ 😖		Goals for tomorrow	The day's score A+ - F 0 = A+, 1-2 = A, 3-4 = A-, 5-6 = B+, 7-9 = B, 10-12 = B-,13-15 = C+ 16-18 = C, 19-21 = C-, 22-24 = D+, 25-27 = D, 28+ = F Your Grade:

Your	A year for change A month for change A week for change A day for change Day 2	**FLog**

Date:	*Don't FLog for temporary improvement,* *FLog for LIFE improvement!*	M T W TH F Sa Su

Sleep	Hours, time, quality, dreams, any A.M. symptoms? Circle a face: 😃 🙂 😐 🙁 😣

Time to eat: **Solid or** **liquid** **Score:**	4am - 11am, List all ingredients, be descriptive but don't over think it.

Symptoms:	How do you feel? See symptoms chart.

Time to eat: **Solid or** **liquid** **Score:**	11am - 4pm, List all ingredients

Symptoms:	How do you feel? See symptoms chart.

Time to eat: **Solid or** **liquid** **Score:**	4pm - 8pm, List all ingredients

Symptoms:	How do you feel? See symptoms chart.
Time to eat: **Solid or** **liquid** **Score:**	8pm - 4am, List all ingredients
Symptoms:	How do you feel? See symptoms chart.

H2O Per 8oz	Exercise, Minutes and type Anaerobic:	Minutes and type Aerobic:	Stool Analysis, time, type and the face you made
Supplements and/ or medication, other medical related logging AM: YES/NO PM: YES/NO			☺ ☺ ☺ ☹ 😣 ☺ ☺ ☺ ☹ 😣 ☺ ☺ ☺ ☹ 😣
Notes, thoughts and goals for the day ☺ ☺ ☺ ☹ 😣		Goals for tomorrow	The day's score A+ - F 0 = A+, 1-2 = A, 3-4 = A-, 5-6 = B+, 7-9 = B, 10-12 = B-,13-15 = C+ 16-18 = C, 19-21 = C-, 22-24 = D+, 25-27 = D, 28+ = F Your Grade:

Your	A year for change A month for change A week for change A day for change Day 3	**FLog**

Date:	*Keep Calm, FLog on!*	M T W TH F Sa Su

Sleep	Hours, time, quality, dreams, any A.M. symptoms? Circle a face: 😃 🙂 😐 🙁 😖

Time to eat: **Solid or** **liquid** **Score:**	4am - 11am, List all ingredients, be descriptive but don't over think it.

Symptoms:	How do you feel? See symptoms chart.

Time to eat: **Solid or** **liquid** **Score:**	11am - 4pm, List all ingredients

Symptoms:	How do you feel? See symptoms chart.

Time to eat: **Solid or** **liquid** **Score:**	4pm - 8pm, List all ingredients

Symptoms:	How do you feel? See symptoms chart.
Time to eat: Solid or liquid	8pm - 4am, List all ingredients
Score:	
Symptoms:	How do you feel? See symptoms chart.

H2O Per 8oz	Exercise, Minutes and type Anaerobic:	Minutes and type Aerobic:	Stool Analysis, time, type and the face you made
Supplements and/ or medication, other medical related logging AM: YES/NO			☺ ☺ ☺ ☹ 😖
			☺ ☺ ☺ ☹ 😖
PM: YES/NO			☺ ☺ ☺ ☹ 😖
Notes, thoughts and goals for the day ☺ ☺ ☺ ☹ 😖		Goals for tomorrow	The day's score A+ - F 0 = A+, 1-2 = A, 3-4 = A-, 5-6 = B+, 7-9 = B, 10-12 = B-,13-15 = C+ 16-18 = C, 19-21 = C-, 22-24 = D+, 25-27 = D, 28+ = F Your Grade:

Your	A year for change A month for change A week for change A day for change Day 4	FLog
Date:	***You're FLogging Awesome!***	M T W TH F Sa Su
Sleep	Hours, time, quality, dreams, any A.M. symptoms? Circle a face: ☺ ☺ ☺ ☹ 😖	
Time to eat: Solid or liquid **Score:**	4am - 11am, List all ingredients, be descriptive but don't over think it.	
Symptoms:	How do you feel? See symptoms chart.	
Time to eat: Solid or liquid **Score:**	11am - 4pm, List all ingredients	
Symptoms:	How do you feel? See symptoms chart.	
Time to eat: Solid or liquid **Score:**	4pm - 8pm, List all ingredients	

Symptoms:	How do you feel? See symptoms chart.
Time to eat: Solid or liquid **Score**:	8pm - 4am, List all ingredients
Symptoms:	How do you feel? See symptoms chart.

H2O Per 8oz	Exercise, Minutes and type Anaerobic:	Minutes and type Aerobic:	Stool Analysis, time, type and the face you made
Supplements and/ or medication, other medical related logging AM: YES/NO PM: YES/NO			😃 🙂 😐 🙁 😖 😃 🙂 😐 🙁 😖 😃 🙂 😐 🙁 😖
Notes, thoughts and goals for the day 😃 🙂 😐 🙁 😖		Goals for tomorrow	The day's score A+ - F 0 = A+, 1-2 = A, 3-4 = A-, 5-6 = B+, 7-9 = B, 10-12 = B-,13-15 = C+ 16-18 = C, 19-21 = C-, 22-24 = D+, 25-27 = D, 28+ = F Your Grade:

Your	A year for change A month for change A week for change A day for change Day 5	FLog

Date:	*To all mankind and our animals, be well and prevent disease in the body. Protect the immune system.*	M T W TH F Sa Su

Sleep	Hours, time, quality, dreams, any A.M. symptoms? Circle a face: 😃 🙂 😐 🙁 😖

Time to eat: **Solid or** **liquid** **Score:**	4am - 11am, List all ingredients, be descriptive but don't over think it.

Symptoms:	How do you feel? See symptoms chart.

Time to eat: **Solid or** **liquid** **Score:**	11am - 4pm, List all ingredients

Symptoms:	How do you feel? See symptoms chart.

Time to eat: **Solid or** **liquid** **Score:**	4pm - 8pm, List all ingredients

Symptoms:	How do you feel? See symptoms chart.
Time to eat: Solid or liquid **Score:**	8pm - 4am, List all ingredients
Symptoms:	How do you feel? See symptoms chart.

H2O Per 8oz	Exercise, Minutes and type Anaerobic:	Minutes and type Aerobic:	Stool Analysis, time, type and the face you made
Supplements and/ or medication, other medical related logging AM: YES/NO PM: YES/NO			🙂 🙂 😐 🙁 😣 🙂 🙂 😐 🙁 😣 🙂 🙂 😐 🙁 😣
Notes, thoughts and goals for the day 🙂 🙂 😐 🙁 😣		Goals for tomorrow	The day's score A+ - F 0 = A+, 1-2 = A, 3-4 = A-, 5-6 = B+, 7-9 = B, 10-12 = B-,13-15 = C+ 16-18 = C, 19-21 = C-, 22-24 = D+, 25-27 = D, 28+ = F Your Grade:

Your	A year for change A month for change A week for change A day for change Day 6	FLog

Date:	*Cruciferous vegetables: Depending on raw or cooked one may be better for your personal digestion (1)*	M T W TH F Sa Su

Sleep	Hours, time, quality, dreams, any A.M. symptoms? Circle a face: 😃 🙂 😐 🙁 😖

Time to eat: Solid or liquid Score:	4am - 11am, List all ingredients, be descriptive but don't over think it.

Symptoms:	How do you feel? See symptoms chart.

Time to eat: Solid or liquid Score:	11am - 4pm, List all ingredients

Symptoms:	How do you feel? See symptoms chart.

Time to eat: Solid or liquid Score:	4pm - 8pm, List all ingredients

Symptoms:	How do you feel? See symptoms chart.
Time to eat: Solid or liquid **Score:**	8pm - 4am, List all ingredients
Symptoms:	How do you feel? See symptoms chart.

H2O Per 8oz	Exercise, Minutes and type Anaerobic:	Minutes and type Aerobic:	Stool Analysis, time, type and the face you made
Supplements and/ or medication, other medical related logging AM: YES/NO PM: YES/NO			😛 🙂 😐 🙁 😖 😛 🙂 😐 🙁 😖 😛 🙂 😐 🙁 😖
Notes, thoughts and goals for the day 😛 🙂 😐 🙁 😖		Goals for tomorrow	The day's score A+ - F 0 = A+, 1-2 = A, 3-4 = A-, 5-6 = B+, 7-9 = B, 10-12 = B-,13-15 = C+ 16-18 = C, 19-21 = C-, 22-24 = D+, 25-27 = D, 28+ = F Your Grade:

Your	A year for change A month for change A week for change A day for change Day 7	FLog

Date:	*Out of my sickness comes wellness!*	M T W TH F Sa Su

Sleep	Hours, time, quality, dreams, any A.M. symptoms? Circle a face: 😃 ☺ 😐 🙁 😖

Time to eat: Solid or liquid	4am - 11am, List all ingredients, be descriptive but don't over think it.
Score:	

Symptoms:	How do you feel? See symptoms chart.

Time to eat: Solid or liquid	11am - 4pm, List all ingredients
Score:	

Symptoms:	How do you feel? See symptoms chart.

Time to eat: Solid or liquid	4pm - 8pm, List all ingredients
Score:	

Symptoms:	How do you feel? See symptoms chart.
Time to eat: Solid or liquid **Score:**	8pm - 4am, List all ingredients
Symptoms:	How do you feel? See symptoms chart.

H2O Per 8oz	Exercise, Minutes and type Anaerobic:	Minutes and type Aerobic:	Stool Analysis, time, type and the face you made
Supplements and/ or medication, other medical related logging AM: YES/NO PM: YES/NO			🙂 🙂 😐 🙁 😖 🙂 🙂 😐 🙁 😖 🙂 🙂 😐 🙁 😖
Notes, thoughts and goals for the day 🙂 🙂 😐 🙁 😖		Goals for tomorrow	The day's score A+ - F 0 = A+, 1-2 = A, 3-4 = A-, 5-6 = B+, 7-9 = B, 10-12 = B-,13-15 = C+ 16-18 = C, 19-21 = C-, 22-24 = D+, 25-27 = D, 28+ = F Your Grade:

Cheat sheet

Water intake goal:	Exercise goal:	Supplements and/ or medication:	Sleep:
Women: 91oz Men: 125oz This really does mean just plain water or a water based non-sugar based liquid like herbal tea	3-4 days a week 20-45minutes Anaerobic, aerobic (cardio) or both	Record that your took them either in the AM or PM. Record any other pertinent information. i.e. if you need to record blood pressure, ketones, blood sugar etc.	Goal 7-8 hours Keep a regular sleep/wake schedule Before sleep, do gentle stretches or meditate 5-10 minutes to fall asleep

Stool Analysis: Goal 3-4	Food law, simple list.	See Food Law pages for detailed food lists	
1 - hard to pass small lumps 2 - lumpy hard sausage like 3 - sausage like with cracks on surface 4 - like a smooth soft sausage 5 - soft blobs with clear edges 6 - mushy consistency with ragged edges 7 - liquid consistency with no solid pieces	**High risk:** Gluten Soy Corn Dairy Legumes Grains Sugar Alternative Sweetners	**Medium Risk:** Nightshades Whey Sheep's milk Food additives NSAIDs Alcohol	**Low Risk:** All eggs Nuts* Seeds* Ghee Stevia Emulsifiers/thickeners FODMAPs

Symptoms	How do you feel?		
Digestive: Diarrhea Constipation Nausea Gas Bloating Cramps Indigestion Burping Cravings Acid reflux Heartburn GERD	**Cognitive/Cerebral:** Headache Migraine Brain fog ADD/ADHD Lack of focus Fatigue Memory loss Anxiety Sleeplessness, Depression Anger Vertigo Hearing loss Vision loss Vision/blurry/spotty/pain	**Hormonal:** Heat flash Mood swing Irregular period PMS Thyroid disfunction Decreased libido Weight gain Infertility Breast tenderness Low muscle mass Heavier/lighter bleeding Back ache cramps	**Body:** Acne Hives Rash itching Sweating Joint pain Muscle ache Gout Arthritis Swelling Numbness/tingling Body/breath odor Dry eye Hair loss High blood pressure

Chapter 1

Playing the Game of Clue

I fell in love with horses as soon as I could sit on one, which was when I was about three years old. Every Christmas and birthday I prayed and begged for a pony, but I never got one. When I was in my early teens, God finally answered my prayers to be around horses. Sadly, it was someone else's misfortune that opened the door into the world of horses for me. Our next door neighbor had been diagnosed with ALS. His wife was my mom's best friend. While he was still able to sit up in a wheelchair, he was taking riding lessons at a therapeutic horsemanship program called R.E.I.N.S, (Riding Emphasizing Individual Needs and Strengths) in North County San Diego. It was through these neighbors that I found out that this very special riding program needed volunteers, which of course I was more than ready and willing to start doing.

From then on I spent almost every Saturday and summer vacation volunteering at R.E.I.N.S. My hard work and leadership earned me the 1999 San Diego County Volunteer of the Year award. At the age of eighteen I was approached by the facility to become a certified instructor. I was honored but very hesitant. At this time in my life I was wondering what I was going to do with my future—I did know that I needed a job—so I accepted and began training for the certification program. Teaching came to me naturally, and I loved it!

For several years I assisted with the riding lessons of a middle aged woman who had Multiple Sclerosis. Being involved in her lessons is when I first noticed that people with MS could have good days and bad days. I knew very little about this disease but I saw first hand how deteriorating it is. Some days this woman would be in a wheelchair and other days she would be walking with the help of a cane. She often cancelled her weekly lesson because she was just simply not up for the trip out to the barn. Her body was frail, she had poor use of her hands, and talked with a slur. One of the most heartbreaking aspects of her story is, that she once had been an avid equestrian, and now she was only able do a walk lesson and use one finger hooked onto the reins to steer the horse.

One of my students was a younger woman at a less progressive stage of MS. Most of the time she was able to drive herself to the lessons. She sometimes used a cane to walk and on some occasions she felt strong enough to walk without it. She had bladder issues and she would even joke about wearing adult diapers. She had a great sense of humor, which I admired, and she really tried hard to just be normal. Up to that point, my understanding of multiple sclerosis was limited to my experiences with these two women. Years later, as my doctor told me my MRI results looked like MS, I thought back to these two ladies. In the past what I had felt was that my only connection with them was our love for horses—boy did that change! Even when the doctors discovered my diagnosis of MS, I *still* did not want to relate to them and I did not want their story to be my story.

I continued to teach through my early twenties at three different facilities and in three different counties. Including a year in Los Angeles teaching at Ride On L.A. (another therapeutic riding program) in Chatsworth CA. I also completed certification as an equine massage therapist. As it turned out, life had other plans for me and in 2005 I found myself back in Los Angeles around the age of twenty-four. Unfortunately, when I returned to L.A. there wasn't another opportunity to teach. Instead, I schooled horses a couple of days a week at Ride On L.A, and I found a great job working full time at Calabasas Saddlery in Calabasas, CA. If I couldn't be with horses all day, then the next best thing was to hang around horse people and help them buy their riding equipment. Working at the saddlery was quite a change from working in the riding arena five days a week. In hindsight, the career change was heaven sent, because I wouldn't have been physically able to teach and ride. I couldn't think of a better way to pay my bills than to be learning another side of the equestrian world.

Everything was going well, until I foolishly used the bottom end of a bucket as a step stool while trying to hang up merchandise. Suddenly, I found myself tipped over and I landed hard on the sharp edge of the store's front counter. My thigh was black and blue in minutes. I finally couldn't tolerate the pain I was having while walking and after seeing an orthopedic surgeon and having an MRI done of my hip, I found out that I had a labral tear. This definitely made sense why I was in so much pain and why riding horses was becoming difficult. My left leg was very weak, and if the horse I was riding quickly decided to go left—I would go right, right into the *dirt*!

After surgery, I noticed that I wasn't regaining full function of my left leg and riding horses was still difficult. This was supposed to have been an easy recovery, yet something wasn't right. I kept wondering if perhaps during surgery they had hit a nerve or cut into a muscle they shouldn't have. I couldn't walk far in flip flops because my toes didn't want to hold on to my sandal, and I couldn't walk far without developing a limp. You know when you shake your foot real fast just out of pure boredom? Well, I couldn't do that either. It was even difficult to cross my second toe over my big toe. When I told the orthopedic surgeon that my leg was very weak, he just sent me for more physical therapy. I attended the physical therapy sessions, but I still felt that my actual symptoms weren't being addressed. I appeared strong and capable, so I graduated physical therapy quickly both times. I began to accept, for whatever reason, that my leg was never going to be the same.

In 2008, I was determined to get a proposal out of my boyfriend (now husband). I finally confronted him about the fact that I was not willing to wait until we had been dating ten or more years to get married. During the very heated discussion, he pulled out a box with the exact ring I had chosen a few months earlier. I was *speechless*. We set the wedding for the following June, because that would be our nine year anniversary and that was as close to ten years as I was willing to get. Now, I was immersed into planning the wedding. At the time, I weighed 198 pounds and, naturally, I wanted to get wedding fit! My solution was a pescatarian diet that made sea food my primary source of animal protein. It worked, and I got down to 170 pounds for the wedding. We pulled off the wedding in the short nine months of planning and it was like a day on the red carpet. Flashing lights and the joy of family and friends celebrating our vows with us—and a great party afterwards.

I had become acclimated to the diet so I kept it up after the wedding. I thought I was pretty healthy, and did as much working out as my left leg could allow. I could run a mile on the treadmill and with some rest and proper stretching, I'd only have a slight limp for the rest of the day. Other symptoms then included fatigue on hot days, feeling like a wet noodle when getting out of a hot bath, and almost passing out after getting out of a jacuzzi. I simply attributed these episodes to not eating enough, which was probably true because I use to half starve myself with my diet.

This was not the first of my odd diet ideas; as a 220 pound teen, I thought the way to lose weight was a diet consisting of lettuce sandwiches with taco bell sauce, alongside the well known over-the-counter supplement Metabolife for energy. Besides iron pills prescribed by my doctor for severe anemia, Metabolife was a miracle for added energy, and I was dependent on it. Between my Jazzercise addiction, riding miles on my rollerblades, and busting my butt out with the horses, I'd say I was a fairly active teen, but with a very poor diet. I managed to lose twenty pounds, but it was the wrong way to do it; *"I mean, lettuce sandwiches, really?"*

I took the Metabolife supplement until I was around twenty-eight. I simply felt that it couldn't possibly be good for me in the long run, so it was time to wean myself off of it and try something else. That being said, at least my pescatarian diet did help maintain my weight and made me feel more energetic. Going "Gluten Free" was a new fad, so I became mostly gluten free after getting married. I definitely wanted to maintain my weight loss and reduce more pounds. I rationalized that my diet was a lifestyle, and some sugar inducing happiness or a little gluten here and there couldn't hurt. It worked for me then, but I was clueless about the damage of inflammation going on under the surface.

My husband and friends knew very well that if I said I needed to pee, they needed to find me a bathroom or a bush *asap* because it would come on so sudden and urgent, that nothing was going to stop it from becoming a dreadful accident. Drinking alcohol only made it worse. "Angela has a pee emergency" became somewhat of a running joke, because what's a better way of dealing with something difficult than finding the humor in it? In retrospect, finding out what was causing those symptoms back then may have prevented more damage. With the help of conventional medicine, there would have been hope of not relapsing—had I known.

Some time around 2010 I began suffering from numbness in my arms so severe that it would wake me up from an otherwise, peaceful sleep. It was excruciatingly painful when one of my arms was dead asleep and began to "wake up". I'd have to get up and walk around or I'd lay there cursing my arm. I eventually taught myself to quiet the spastic and cramping muscles in my left leg by foam rolling. I had also suffered from sleep paralysis since I was a child, but I mostly ignored it since it happened very seldom. I remember around the age of thirteen, I felt brave enough to tell my aunt, who was a nurse, how I couldn't move or open my eyes to wake up. She was not familiar with the symptom and could not recommend anything. I simply did not make a big enough fuss about it, so it was never addressed. But as far as those early problematic symptoms, I had been in denial, and did not believe they warranted a visit to the doctor. Denial is a big monster, but it can feel much more comfortable than facing scary issues.

Sometimes I wish my parents had been hippies who grew and harvested all our produce, raised our own animals for food, and that those animals also only ate what nature intended them to eat. I wish we had stayed away from processed foods and fast food. As a child my skin was blotchy and confused on which color it wanted to be. When I was about sixteen years old I was so anemic I could barely manage getting down the stairs. The doctors only asked if I had heavy periods. For years, I took iron pills which helped with the anemia. My skin got better as I grew but sometimes it flared—I always thought I was allergic to the sun. If you saw a picture of me at the age of ten, you might not be able to recognize me because of the splotchy condition of my skin and my young overweight body.

They were not hippies, and although we had a garden, they still bought us fast food, pizza, hot dogs on buns and fish sticks. I understand that my parents were very busy, and this way of eating was both a matter of convenience and a way to placate us kids that often begged for those foods. Still, my diet growing up was probably better than today's Standard American Diet. I certainly had a mother and grandmother with good home cooking skills. There were definitely some ingredients and foods they could have omitted, if only they had known of their inflammatory nature.

My parents are wonderful and I am very blessed, but they simply didn't know any better. I strongly urge men and women to try to be as healthy as they can be before having a child, so that child has a fighting chance against the harsh environment we live in today. The world has changed drastically in so short a time, much faster than our bodies can adapt. I also urge parents to take strong roles in their family's health. We'll be fortunate if our parents are around a long time and experience a full and healthy golden era. However, they have to decide for themselves to be their healthiest.

Your	A year for change A month for change A week for change A day for change Day 8	**FLog**

Date:	*FLogLife*	M T W TH F Sa Su

Sleep	Hours, time, quality, dreams, any A.M. symptoms? Circle a face: ☺ ☺ 😐 ☹ 😖

Time to eat: Solid or liquid	4am - 11am, List all ingredients, be descriptive but don't over think it.

Score:

Symptoms:	How do you feel? See symptoms chart.

Time to eat: Solid or liquid	11am - 4pm, List all ingredients

Score:

Symptoms:	How do you feel? See symptoms chart.

Time to eat: Solid or liquid	4pm - 8pm, List all ingredients

Score:

Symptoms:	How do you feel? See symptoms chart.
Time to eat: Solid or liquid **Score:**	8pm - 4am, List all ingredients
Symptoms:	How do you feel? See symptoms chart.

H2O Per 8oz	Exercise, Minutes and type Anaerobic:	Minutes and type Aerobic:	Stool Analysis, time, type and the face you made
Supplements and/ or medication, other medical related logging AM: YES/NO PM: YES/NO			☺ ☺ 😐 ☹ 😖 ☺ ☺ 😐 ☹ 😖 ☺ ☺ 😐 ☹ 😖
Notes, thoughts and goals for the day ☺ ☺ 😐 ☹ 😖		Goals for tomorrow	The day's score A+ - F 0 = A+, 1-2 = A, 3-4 = A-, 5-6 = B+, 7-9 = B, 10-12 = B-,13-15 = C+ 16-18 = C, 19-21 = C-, 22-24 = D+, 25-27 = D, 28+ = F Your Grade:

Your	A year for change A month for change A week for change A day for change Day 9	FLog

Date:	***Make it FLogalicious***	M T W TH F Sa Su

Sleep	Hours, time, quality, dreams, any A.M. symptoms? Circle a face: 😃 ☺ 😐 ☹ 😖

Time to eat: Solid or liquid **Score:**	4am - 11am, List all ingredients, be descriptive but don't over think it.

Symptoms:	How do you feel? See symptoms chart.

Time to eat: Solid or liquid **Score:**	11am - 4pm, List all ingredients

Symptoms:	How do you feel? See symptoms chart.

Time to eat: Solid or liquid **Score:**	4pm - 8pm, List all ingredients

Symptoms:	How do you feel? See symptoms chart.
Time to eat: Solid or liquid **Score:**	8pm - 4am, List all ingredients
Symptoms:	How do you feel? See symptoms chart.

H2O Per 8oz	Exercise, Minutes and type Anaerobic:	Minutes and type Aerobic:	Stool Analysis, time, type and the face you made
Supplements and/ or medication, other medical related logging AM: YES/NO PM: YES/NO			😀 🙂 😐 🙁 😣 😀 🙂 😐 🙁 😣 😀 🙂 😐 🙁 😣
Notes, thoughts and goals for the day 😀 🙂 😐 🙁 😣		Goals for tomorrow	The day's score A+ - F 0 = A+, 1-2 = A, 3-4 = A-, 5-6 = B+, 7-9 = B, 10-12 = B-,13-15 = C+ 16-18 = C, 19-21 = C-, 22-24 = D+, 25-27 = D, 28+ = F Your Grade:

Your	<u>A year for change A month for change A week for change A day for change</u> Day 10	**FLog**

Date:	*Create your body's unique diet*	M T W TH F Sa Su

Sleep	Hours, time, quality, dreams, any A.M. symptoms? Circle a face: ☺ ☺ ☺ ☹ 😖

Time to eat: Solid or liquid	4am - 11am, List all ingredients, be descriptive but don't over think it.
Score:	

Symptoms:	How do you feel? See symptoms chart.

Time to eat: Solid or liquid	11am - 4pm, List all ingredients
Score:	

Symptoms:	How do you feel? See symptoms chart.

Time to eat: Solid or liquid	4pm - 8pm, List all ingredients
Score:	

Symptoms:	How do you feel? See symptoms chart.
Time to eat: Solid or liquid	8pm - 4am, List all ingredients
Score:	
Symptoms:	How do you feel? See symptoms chart.

H2O Per 8oz	Exercise, Minutes and type Anaerobic:	Minutes and type Aerobic:	Stool Analysis, time, type and the face you made
Supplements and/ or medication, other medical related logging AM: YES/NO			☺ ☺ ☺ ☹ 😖
			☺ ☺ ☺ ☹ 😖
PM: YES/NO			☺ ☺ ☺ ☹ 😖
Notes, thoughts and goals for the day ☺ ☺ ☺ ☹ 😖		Goals for tomorrow	The day's score A+ - F

0 = A+, 1-2 = A, 3-4 = A-, 5-6 = B+, 7-9 = B, 10-12 = B-,13-15 = C+ 16-18 = C, 19-21 = C-, 22-24 = D+, 25-27 = D, 28+ = F

Your Grade: |

Your	A year for change A month for change A week for change A day for change Day 11	**FLog**

Date:	***You don't have to have a vegan, primal or paleo lifestyle to FLog! Follow the Food Law***	M T W TH F Sa Su

Sleep	Hours, time, quality, dreams, any A.M. symptoms? Circle a face: 😃 ☺ 😐 🙁 😖

Time to eat: Solid or liquid	4am - 11am, List all ingredients, be descriptive but don't over think it.
Score:	

Symptoms:	How do you feel? See symptoms chart.

Time to eat: Solid or liquid	11am - 4pm, List all ingredients
Score:	

Symptoms:	How do you feel? See symptoms chart.

Time to eat: Solid or liquid	4pm - 8pm, List all ingredients
Score:	

Symptoms:	How do you feel? See symptoms chart.
Time to eat: Solid or liquid **Score:**	8pm - 4am, List all ingredients
Symptoms:	How do you feel? See symptoms chart.

H2O Per 8oz	Exercise, Minutes and type Anaerobic:	Minutes and type Aerobic:	Stool Analysis, time, type and the face you made
Supplements and/ or medication, other medical related logging AM: YES/NO PM: YES/NO			😀 🙂 😐 🙁 😖 😀 🙂 😐 🙁 😖 😀 🙂 😐 🙁 😖
Notes, thoughts and goals for the day 😀 🙂 😐 🙁 😖		Goals for tomorrow	The day's score A+ - F 0 = A+, 1-2 = A, 3-4 = A-, 5-6 = B+, 7-9 = B, 10-12 = B-,13-15 = C+ 16-18 = C, 19-21 = C-, 22-24 = D+, 25-27 = D, 28+ = F Your Grade:

Your	A year for change A month for change A week for change A day for change Day 12	**FLog**

Date:	*Cows are the biggest methane producers, which breaks down our ozone! Stop the over production of beef. Eat less or zero! (2)*	M T W TH F Sa Su

Sleep	Hours, time, quality, dreams, any A.M. symptoms? Circle a face: 😃 🙂 😐 🙁 😖

Time to eat: Solid or liquid **Score:**	4am - 11am, List all ingredients, be descriptive but don't over think it.

Symptoms:	How do you feel? See symptoms chart.

Time to eat: Solid or liquid **Score:**	11am - 4pm, List all ingredients

Symptoms:	How do you feel? See symptoms chart.

Time to eat: Solid or liquid **Score:**	4pm - 8pm, List all ingredients

Symptoms:	How do you feel? See symptoms chart.
Time to eat: Solid or liquid **Score:**	8pm - 4am, List all ingredients
Symptoms:	How do you feel? See symptoms chart.

H2O Per 8oz	Exercise, Minutes and type Anaerobic:	Minutes and type Aerobic:	Stool Analysis, time, type and the face you made
Supplements and/ or medication, other medical related logging AM: YES/NO PM: YES/NO			😀 🙂 😐 🙁 😣 😀 🙂 😐 🙁 😣 😀 🙂 😐 🙁 😣
Notes, thoughts and goals for the day 😀 🙂 😐 🙁 😣		Goals for tomorrow	The day's score A+ - F 0 = A+, 1-2 = A, 3-4 = A-, 5-6 = B+, 7-9 = B, 10-12 = B-,13-15 = C+ 16-18 = C, 19-21 = C-, 22-24 = D+, 25-27 = D, 28+ = F Your Grade:

Your	A year for change A month for change A week for change A day for change Day 13	**FLog**

Date:	*You're body is the judge of your intake.* *What are you putting in you mouth today?*	M T W TH F Sa Su

Sleep	Hours, time, quality, dreams, any A.M. symptoms? Circle a face: 😁 ☺ 😐 ☹ 😣

Time to eat: **Solid or** **liquid** **Score:**	4am - 11am, List all ingredients, be descriptive but don't over think it.

Symptoms:	How do you feel? See symptoms chart.

Time to eat: **Solid or** **liquid** **Score:**	11am - 4pm, List all ingredients

Symptoms:	How do you feel? See symptoms chart.

Time to eat: **Solid or** **liquid** **Score:**	4pm - 8pm, List all ingredients

Symptoms:	How do you feel? See symptoms chart.
Time to eat: Solid or liquid	8pm - 4am, List all ingredients
Score:	
Symptoms:	How do you feel? See symptoms chart.

H2O Per 8oz	Exercise, Minutes and type Anaerobic:	Minutes and type Aerobic:	Stool Analysis, time, type and the face you made
Supplements and/ or medication, other medical related logging AM: YES/NO			🙂 🙂 😐 🙁 😣 🙂 🙂 😐 🙁 😣 🙂 🙂 😐 🙁 😣
PM: YES/NO			
Notes, thoughts and goals for the day 🙂 🙂 😐 🙁 😣		Goals for tomorrow	The day's score A+ - F 0 = A+, 1-2 = A, 3-4 = A-, 5-6 = B+, 7-9 = B, 10-12 = B-,13-15 = C+ 16-18 = C, 19-21 = C-, 22-24 = D+, 25-27 = D, 28+ = F Your Grade:

Your	A year for change A month for change A week for change A day for change Day 14	**FLog**

Date:	*It is sown a natural body, it is raised a spiritual body. If there is a natural body, there is also a spiritual body 1 Cor. 15:44*	M T W TH F Sa Su

Sleep	Hours, time, quality, dreams, any A.M. symptoms? Circle a face: 😃 ☺ 😐 ☹ 😖

Time to eat: Solid or liquid **Score:**	4am - 11am, List all ingredients, be descriptive but don't over think it.

Symptoms:	How do you feel? See symptoms chart.

Time to eat: Solid or liquid **Score:**	11am - 4pm, List all ingredients

Symptoms:	How do you feel? See symptoms chart.

Time to eat: Solid or liquid **Score:**	4pm - 8pm, List all ingredients

Symptoms:	How do you feel? See symptoms chart.
Time to eat: Solid or liquid **Score:**	8pm - 4am, List all ingredients
Symptoms:	How do you feel? See symptoms chart.

H2O Per 8oz	Exercise, Minutes and type Anaerobic:	Minutes and type Aerobic:	Stool Analysis, time, type and the face you made
Supplements and/ or medication, other medical related logging AM: YES/NO PM: YES/NO			😀 🙂 😐 🙁 😖 😀 🙂 😐 🙁 😖 😀 🙂 😐 🙁 😖
Notes, thoughts and goals for the day 😀 🙂 😐 🙁 😖		Goals for tomorrow	The day's score A+ - F 0 = A+, 1-2 = A, 3-4 = A-, 5-6 = B+, 7-9 = B, 10-12 = B-,13-15 = C+ 16-18 = C, 19-21 = C-, 22-24 = D+, 25-27 = D, 28+ = F Your Grade:

Cheat sheet

Water intake goal:	Exercise goal:	Supplements and/ or medication:	Sleep:
Women: 91oz Men: 125oz This really does mean just plain water or a water based non-sugar based liquid like herbal tea	3-4 days a week 20-45minutes Anaerobic, aerobic (cardio) or both	Record that your took them either in the AM or PM. Record any other pertinent information. i.e. if you need to record blood pressure, ketones, blood sugar etc.	Goal 7-8 hours Keep a regular sleep/ wake schedule Before sleep, do gentle stretches or meditate 5-10 minutes to fall asleep

Stool Analysis: Goal 3-4	Food law, simple list.	See Food Law pages for detailed food lists	
1 - hard to pass small lumps 2 - lumpy hard sausage like 3 - sausage like with cracks on surface 4 - like a smooth soft sausage 5 - soft blobs with clear edges 6 - mushy consistency with ragged edges 7 - liquid consistency with no solid pieces	**High risk:** Gluten Soy Corn Dairy Legumes Grains Sugar Alternative Sweetners	**Medium Risk:** Nightshades Whey Sheep's milk Food additives NSAIDs Alcohol	**Low Risk:** All eggs Nuts* Seeds* Ghee Stevia Emulsifiers/thickeners FODMAPs

Symptoms	How do you feel?		
Digestive: Diarrhea Constipation Nausea Gas Bloating Cramps Indigestion Burping Cravings Acid reflux Heartburn GERD	**Cognitive/Cerebral:** Headache Migraine Brain fog ADD/ ADHD Lack of focus Fatigue Memory loss Anxiety Sleeplessness, Depression Anger Vertigo Hearing loss Vision loss Vision/ blurry/spotty/pain	**Hormonal:** Heat flash Mood swing Irregular period PMS Thyroid disfunction Decreased libido Weight gain Infertility Breast tenderness Low muscle mass Heavier/ lighter bleeding Back ache cramps	**Body:** Acne Hives Rash itching Sweating Joint pain Muscle ache Gout Arthritis Swelling Numbness/ tingling Body/breath odor Dry eye Hair loss High blood pressure

MY JOURNEY

Chapter 2

A Whole Mess of Changes

As an equine massage therapist I worked with a horse or two each year. A wonderful friend suggested that I massage people. I had never been motivated enough to work on people because I questioned, "How would it feel working on a person rather than an animal?" Yet once I did it, I liked it. *A lot!* I began to pursue formal education in the field of massage in 2011, and around the age of 30 I began to start a new career path. Unfortunately, that new career path took me further from riding because there simply was not enough time to ride, and the joy was not the same because of my left leg's challenges. I slowly stopped riding altogether.

After graduating from massage school and beginning a second job as a massage therapist during the summer of 2012, I was trying to fill my water bottle when I noticed I couldn't hold it still with my left hand. I found it somewhat strange, but at the time I did not worry too much because the day before I had hit my left elbow really hard on the refrigerator door handle. I was sure it was just a pinched nerve that would heal on its own. I felt like I had it under control, but really, and unbeknownst to me, a perfect storm had just raged in my body.

Despite the tremor, I went on with my work at the Saddlery and as a massage therapist as if nothing was wrong. In reality, I was terrified of my weaknesses being exposed. My job at the Saddlery forced me to confront that fear. I could only use the register with one hand and had to ask for assistance when bagging merchandise. Most of the customers had known me for years, but I couldn't bring myself to tell them why I needed help and why these simple tasks were so difficult. I would eventually show some of my co-workers who I was close with, how I couldn't put a pen cap on a pen or staple paper without somehow anchoring my left arm to make it work. Most of these co-workers had even been in my wedding party, so I felt comfortable confiding in them and asking for their help. When I was on my own, simple everyday tasks like driving, using the turn signals, rolling down the window, or turning on the wiper blades were a challenge—because they all required my left side to function. Chopping vegetables was *sure* interesting!

My first job as a massage therapist was at a chiropractor's office. I was in high demand, so I simply tried to cover up the fact that I had a tremor. I would tell clients that it was a unique technique which helped with going against the muscle fibers. Most clients thought it was a cool technique—which it is, especially when I do it on purpose with my right elbow. But as far as my left arm, I just kept that secret to myself. After some time had passed and I felt more comfortable and rather concerned, I finally asked the chiropractor I worked for to look at my left arm. All he needed to do was to take one look at how I couldn't hold my arm straight out in front of me without it shaking. He immediately told me I needed a brain MRI as soon as possible. I was in disbelief. As far as I was concerned, this was still just a pinched nerve—albeit one that was taking way too much time to heal on its own.

At this time, I did not have a full time job that provided health insurance benefits anymore. I was working part time at the saddlery, part time massaging at two locations, and juggling my private clients. Fortunately, we had insurance through my husband's law school health care plan. I didn't even have a general practitioner set up yet, but I got one fast. I was still in denial when I went to my first doctor's appointment, telling myself (and the doctor) that I was there because of a mysterious rash on my skin that was starting to become a major problem.

Thankfully, I was able to schedule an appointment with a neurologist within a few weeks. This doctor checked my reflexes and the sensory nerves on my hands and feet. She made me try to touch my left finger tip to her hand and then back to my nose. I failed on the left side. I barely touched her finger and poked myself in the eye more than my nose. I walked back and forth in the little square room and answered a bunch of routine questions. She actually asked if I was on disability because of the tremor. I responded, "Of course not, I actually believe my job helps my body stay fit and requires my arm to work, where maybe I would favor it if I was not demanding it to perform." Little did I know at the time how true that statement was. When I told her of the refrigerator door handle incident, she set up a nerve conduction test, which confirmed my theory about the pinched nerve. I was quite impressed with my self-diagnostic skills.

At this point, I still couldn't figure out what was wrong with my skin. I also practically was having panic attacks as a massage therapist. Working in a tiny rectangular room with no windows, repetitive music and little light was freaking me out. In addition, sometimes my clients vented to me about their stress issues. It was very difficult to concentrate on myself, working the person's muscles, and listen to them all at once. In retrospect, there were red flags all over that my brain was having trouble multitasking and computing information. In the meantime, I had seen two dermatologists who prescribed steroid creams that did not help the rashes on my skin at all. My hands would eventually crack open in almost every crevice. My forearms had large plaques, and my elbows always felt like they were on fire. I had to wear arm sleeves even in the summer, just to keep them protected. It was painful to rest my arms on anything and I was too embarrassed for people to see them, so I kept them covered.

One doctor said it was psoriasis, but I knew it was nowhere near normal psoriasis. I called it, "Crazy!" I even told one doctor that I thought I was allergic to tomatoes or carrots because eating red sauce or drinking my daily homemade vegetable juice smoothie irritated the rashes. In reality, I had no clue what was wrong and no doctor could resolve it, so I just kept going on as if everything was normal.

Going in for the MRI's, were some of the scariest experiences of my life. I've always been a calm person, so I declined a prescription for valium and slid into the tube. There were loud banging noises, and the earplugs hardly helped. I did not know if this was normal, or how long I would be stuck in that tube. I told myself to close my eyes, breathe, and imagine being in outer space looking at the stars. As awful as this experience was, it was nowhere near as distressing as the phone call I got the next day from my general practitioner: "Well this looks like Multiple Sclerosis, I am so sorry," he said. I was in shock and disbelief, but I remained calm and collected while on the phone. I then scheduled my next appointment with the neurologist. I did not know what to expect or what would happen next. I knew what MS was and how debilitating it could be, because of those two dear ladies I had taught years earlier. Yet, this wasn't my official diagnosis…so what was to come?

I had to go through multiple neurologists, MRI's, and a spinal tap from hell before I got the stamp on my medical record: *Possible* Remitting Remission Multiple Sclerosis. I knew this was where my path had been leading me. I was officially diagnosed with multiple sclerosis in the Spring of 2013 after a few more tests and information gathering. It was tough. I was a new massage therapist trying to make a name for myself, working three jobs, and my husband had just started law school. All of this put a lot of stress on myself, mentally and physically and of course, my marriage. I have heard that stress can be a factor in an MS relapse, which may have been the start of the tremor and increased deterioration of my left leg.

Your	<u>A year for change A month for change A week for change A day for change</u> Day 15	**FLog**

Date:	***Don't get stuck with name it, blame it, tame it prescription pad medicine. Instead find a doctor willing to investigate the causes of your complaint, sickness or disease.***	M T W TH F Sa Su
Sleep	Hours, time, quality, dreams, any A.M. symptoms? Circle a face: 😃 ☺ 😐 🙁 😖	
Time to eat: **Solid or** **liquid** **Score:**	4am - 11am, List all ingredients, be descriptive but don't over think it.	
Symptoms:	How do you feel? See symptoms chart.	
Time to eat: **Solid or** **liquid** **Score:**	11am - 4pm, List all ingredients	
Symptoms:	How do you feel? See symptoms chart.	
Time to eat: **Solid or** **liquid** **Score:**	4pm - 8pm, List all ingredients	

Symptoms:	How do you feel? See symptoms chart.
Time to eat: Solid or liquid **Score:**	8pm - 4am, List all ingredients
Symptoms:	How do you feel? See symptoms chart.

H2O Per 8oz	Exercise, Minutes and type Anaerobic:	Minutes and type Aerobic:	Stool Analysis, time, type and the face you made
Supplements and/ or medication, other medical related logging AM: YES/NO PM: YES/NO			☺ ☺ 😐 ☹ 😖 ☺ ☺ 😐 ☹ 😖 ☺ ☺ 😐 ☹ 😖
Notes, thoughts and goals for the day ☺ ☺ 😐 ☹ 😖		Goals for tomorrow	The day's score A+ - F 0 = A+, 1-2 = A, 3-4 = A-, 5-6 = B+, 7-9 = B, 10-12 = B-,13-15 = C+ 16-18 = C, 19-21 = C-, 22-24 = D+, 25-27 = D, 28+ = F Your Grade:

Your	A year for change A month for change A week for change A day for change Day 16	FLog

Date:	*FLog your diet into shape!*	M T W TH F Sa Su

Sleep	Hours, time, quality, dreams, any A.M. symptoms? Circle a face: ☺ ☺ ☺ ☹ ☣

Time to eat: Solid or liquid	4am - 11am, List all ingredients, be descriptive but don't over think it.
Score:	

Symptoms:	How do you feel? See symptoms chart.

Time to eat: Solid or liquid	11am - 4pm, List all ingredients
Score:	

Symptoms:	How do you feel? See symptoms chart.

Time to eat: Solid or liquid	4pm - 8pm, List all ingredients
Score:	

Symptoms:	How do you feel? See symptoms chart.
Time to eat: Solid or liquid	8pm - 4am, List all ingredients
Score:	
Symptoms:	How do you feel? See symptoms chart.

H2O Per 8oz	Exercise, Minutes and type Anaerobic:	Minutes and type Aerobic:	Stool Analysis, time, type and the face you made
Supplements and/ or medication, other medical related logging AM: YES/NO			☺ ☺ ☺ ☹ 😖
			☺ ☺ ☺ ☹ 😖
PM: YES/NO			☺ ☺ ☺ ☹ 😖
Notes, thoughts and goals for the day ☺ ☺ ☺ ☹ 😖		Goals for tomorrow	The day's score A+ - F 0 = A+, 1-2 = A, 3-4 = A-, 5-6 = B+, 7-9 = B, 10-12 = B-,13-15 = C+ 16-18 = C, 19-21 = C-, 22-24 = D+, 25-27 = D, 28+ = F Your Grade:

Your	A year for change A month for change A week for change A day for change Day 17	FLog

Date:	*Come on little FLoggie, you can choose well today!*	M T W TH F Sa Su

Sleep	Hours, time, quality, dreams, any A.M. symptoms? Circle a face: 😆 🙂 😐 🙁 😖

Time to eat: Solid or liquid Score:	4am - 11am, List all ingredients, be descriptive but don't over think it.

Symptoms:	How do you feel? See symptoms chart.

Time to eat: Solid or liquid Score:	11am - 4pm, List all ingredients

Symptoms:	How do you feel? See symptoms chart.

Time to eat: Solid or liquid Score:	4pm - 8pm, List all ingredients

Symptoms:	How do you feel? See symptoms chart.
Time to eat: Solid or liquid	8pm - 4am, List all ingredients
Score:	
Symptoms:	How do you feel? See symptoms chart.

H2O Per 8oz	Exercise, Minutes and type Anaerobic:	Minutes and type Aerobic:	Stool Analysis, time, type and the face you made
Supplements and/ or medication, other medical related logging AM: YES/NO PM: YES/NO			🙂 🙂 😐 🙁 😖 🙂 🙂 😐 🙁 😖 🙂 🙂 😐 🙁 😖
Notes, thoughts and goals for the day 🙂 🙂 😐 🙁 😖		Goals for tomorrow	The day's score A+ - F 0 = A+, 1-2 = A, 3-4 = A-, 5-6 = B+, 7-9 = B, 10-12 = B-,13-15 = C+ 16-18 = C, 19-21 = C-, 22-24 = D+, 25-27 = D, 28+ = F Your Grade:

Your	A year for change A month for change A week for change A day for change Day 18	FLog

Date:	*Your food plays a huge role on your hormones. Your food effects your mood! (3)*	M T W TH F Sa Su

Sleep	Hours, time, quality, dreams, any A.M. symptoms? Circle a face: ☺ ☺ 😐 🙁 😖

Time to eat: Solid or liquid Score:	4am - 11am, List all ingredients, be descriptive but don't over think it.

Symptoms:	How do you feel? See symptoms chart.

Time to eat: Solid or liquid Score:	11am - 4pm, List all ingredients

Symptoms:	How do you feel? See symptoms chart.

Time to eat: Solid or liquid Score:	4pm - 8pm, List all ingredients

Symptoms:	How do you feel? See symptoms chart.
Time to eat: Solid or liquid **Score:**	8pm - 4am, List all ingredients
Symptoms:	How do you feel? See symptoms chart.

H2O Per 8oz	Exercise, Minutes and type Anaerobic:	Minutes and type Aerobic:	Stool Analysis, time, type and the face you made
Supplements and/ or medication, other medical related logging AM: YES/NO PM: YES/NO			☺ ☺ 😐 ☹ 😖 ☺ ☺ 😐 ☹ 😖 ☺ ☺ 😐 ☹ 😖
Notes, thoughts and goals for the day ☺ ☺ 😐 ☹ 😖		Goals for tomorrow	The day's score A+ - F 0 = A+, 1-2 = A, 3-4 = A-, 5-6 = B+, 7-9 = B, 10-12 = B-,13-15 = C+ 16-18 = C, 19-21 = C-, 22-24 = D+, 25-27 = D, 28+ = F Your Grade:

Your	A year for change A month for change A week for change A day for change Day 19	**FLog**

Date:	*You have a super hero self! Feed your inner super systems.* *Digestive! Immune! Cerebral! Endocrine!*	M T W TH F Sa Su

Sleep	Hours, time, quality, dreams, any A.M. symptoms? Circle a face: ☺ ☺ 😐 ☹ 😖
Time to eat: Solid or liquid **Score:**	4am - 11am, List all ingredients, be descriptive but don't over think it.
Symptoms:	How do you feel? See symptoms chart.
Time to eat: Solid or liquid **Score:**	11am - 4pm, List all ingredients
Symptoms:	How do you feel? See symptoms chart.
Time to eat: Solid or liquid **Score:**	4pm - 8pm, List all ingredients

Symptoms:	How do you feel? See symptoms chart.
Time to eat: **Solid or** **liquid** **Score:**	8pm - 4am, List all ingredients
Symptoms:	How do you feel? See symptoms chart.

H2O Per 8oz	Exercise, Minutes and type Anaerobic:	Minutes and type Aerobic:	Stool Analysis, time, type and the face you made
Supplements and/ or medication, other medical related logging AM: YES/NO PM: YES/NO			😀 ☺ 😐 ☹ 😖 😀 ☺ 😐 ☹ 😖 😀 ☺ 😐 ☹ 😖
Notes, thoughts and goals for the day 😀 ☺ 😐 ☹ 😖		Goals for tomorrow	The day's score A+ - F 0 = A+, 1-2 = A, 3-4 = A-, 5-6 = B+, 7-9 = B, 10-12 = B-,13-15 = C+ 16-18 = C, 19-21 = C-, 22-24 = D+, 25-27 = D, 28+ = F Your Grade:

Your	<u>A year for change A month for change A week for change A day for change</u> Day 20	**FLog**

Date:	***Feel fine today? Well, that's not good enough! Make changes to feel amazing!***	M T W TH F Sa Su

Sleep	Hours, time, quality, dreams, any A.M. symptoms? Circle a face: 😃 🙂 😐 🙁 😫

Time to eat: **Solid or** **liquid** **Score:**	4am - 11am, List all ingredients, be descriptive but don't over think it.

Symptoms:	How do you feel? See symptoms chart.

Time to eat: **Solid or** **liquid** **Score:**	11am - 4pm, List all ingredients

Symptoms:	How do you feel? See symptoms chart.

Time to eat: **Solid or** **liquid** **Score:**	4pm - 8pm, List all ingredients

Symptoms:	How do you feel? See symptoms chart.
Time to eat: Solid or liquid **Score:**	8pm - 4am, List all ingredients
Symptoms:	How do you feel? See symptoms chart.

H2O Per 8oz	Exercise, Minutes and type Anaerobic:	Minutes and type Aerobic:	Stool Analysis, time, type and the face you made
Supplements and/ or medication, other medical related logging AM: YES/NO PM: YES/NO			☺ ☺ ☺ ☹ 😫 ☺ ☺ ☺ ☹ 😫 ☺ ☺ ☺ ☹ 😫
Notes, thoughts and goals for the day ☺ ☺ ☺ ☹ 😫		Goals for tomorrow	The day's score A+ - F 0 = A+, 1-2 = A, 3-4 = A-, 5-6 = B+, 7-9 = B, 10-12 = B-,13-15 = C+ 16-18 = C, 19-21 = C-, 22-24 = D+, 25-27 = D, 28+ = F Your Grade:

ANGELA M. LANDEROS

Your	A year for change A month for change A week for change A day for change Day 21	FLog

Date:	*Eat. Sleep. Poop. Move. FLog.*	M T W TH F Sa Su

Sleep	Hours, time, quality, dreams, any A.M. symptoms? Circle a face: ☺ ☺ ☺ ☹ 😣

Time to eat: Solid or liquid ... Score:	4am - 11am, List all ingredients, be descriptive but don't over think it.

Symptoms:	How do you feel? See symptoms chart.

Time to eat: Solid or liquid ... Score:	11am - 4pm, List all ingredients

Symptoms:	How do you feel? See symptoms chart.

Time to eat: Solid or liquid ... Score:	4pm - 8pm, List all ingredients

112

Symptoms:	How do you feel? See symptoms chart.
Time to eat: Solid or liquid **Score:**	8pm - 4am, List all ingredients
Symptoms:	How do you feel? See symptoms chart.

H2O Per 8oz	Exercise, Minutes and type Anaerobic:	Minutes and type Aerobic:	Stool Analysis, time, type and the face you made
Supplements and/ or medication, other medical related logging AM: YES/NO PM: YES/NO			☺ ☺ ☺ ☹ 😣 ☺ ☺ ☺ ☹ 😣 ☺ ☺ ☺ ☹ 😣
Notes, thoughts and goals for the day ☺ ☺ ☺ ☹ 😣		Goals for tomorrow	The day's score A+ - F 0 = A+, 1-2 = A, 3-4 = A-, 5-6 = B+, 7-9 = B, 10-12 = B-,13-15 = C+ 16-18 = C, 19-21 = C-, 22-24 = D+, 25-27 = D, 28+ = F Your Grade:

Cheat sheet

Water intake goal:	Exercise goal:	Supplements and/or medication:	Sleep:
Women: 91oz Men: 125oz This really does mean just plain water or a water based non-sugar based liquid like herbal tea	3-4 days a week 20-45minutes Anaerobic, aerobic (cardio) or both	Record that your took them either in the AM or PM. Record any other pertinent information. i.e. if you need to record blood pressure, ketones, blood sugar etc.	Goal 7-8 hours Keep a regular sleep/ wake schedule Before sleep, do gentle stretches or meditate 5-10 minutes to fall asleep

Stool Analysis: Goal 3-4	Food law, simple list.	See Food Law pages for detailed food lists	
1 - hard to pass small lumps 2 - lumpy hard sausage like 3 - sausage like with cracks on surface 4 - like a smooth soft sausage 5 - soft blobs with clear edges 6 - mushy consistency with ragged edges 7 - liquid consistency with no solid pieces	**High risk:** Gluten Soy Corn Dairy Legumes Grains Sugar Alternative Sweetners	**Medium Risk:** Nightshades Whey Sheep's milk Food additives NSAIDs Alcohol	**Low Risk:** All eggs Nuts* Seeds* Ghee Stevia Emulsifiers/thickeners FODMAPs

Symptoms	How do you feel?		
Digestive: Diarrhea Constipation Nausea Gas Bloating Cramps Indigestion Burping Cravings Acid reflux Heartburn GERD	**Cognitive/Cerebral:** Headache Migraine Brain fog ADD/ ADHD Lack of focus Fatigue Memory loss Anxiety Sleeplessness, Depression Anger Vertigo Hearing loss Vision loss Vision/ blurry/spotty/pain	**Hormonal:** Heat flash Mood swing Irregular period PMS Thyroid disfunction Decreased libido Weight gain Infertility Breast tenderness Low muscle mass Heavier/ lighter bleeding Back ache cramps	**Body:** Acne Hives Rash itching Sweating Joint pain Muscle ache Gout Arthritis Swelling Numbness/ tingling Body/breath odor Dry eye Hair loss High blood pressure

Chapter 3

Relationships tested

That same summer when my skin had only a few small red itchy spots on my arms, my husband and I moved into a new apartment. I could barely help him and my Dad with all the moving because my left leg was dragging and my mind wanted to explode. My husband and I were working on our marriage with counseling at church. With all these changes and with him in law school, we were not given much time to spend together and it weighed heavy on us. I had a fall out with one of my closest friends, but when my husband was not able to be there, she turned out to be the one who stood by me through every scary neurologist appointment, MRI, spinal tap, and series of IV infusions. She held my hand when I thought I would fall in heels in a nightclub, and held it even tighter for the scary medical procedures with doctors. Thank you Devon! I'll love you forever!

Halfway through my husband's first year of law school, he discovered the school offered a study abroad summer program in Mexico. It happened to be in the area where his Dad and other immediate family live, and where he spent part of his childhood. He was very excited about it, but I wasn't going to tell him that I thought he was crazy because I was in the middle of getting diagnosed with MS, and had many more scary doctor appointments yet to come. I was terrified of him leaving, but I couldn't say that to him. It was a great opportunity, and how could he pass it up. Sure enough, when summer came he left for seven weeks, I fortunately had Devon, who was more than happy to accompany me to all of those appointments. Although, she did have to miss a lot of work. She also worked at the Saddlery and thankfully they completely understood the situation in order to give her the time off.

I had to get a passport to join him his last week in Mexico. This was the most symptomatic time of my life and I didn't even know 100% what was wrong with me. I left the country wondering why my right eye felt like I had been in a fist fight. The weather in Mexico was hot, and I looked a bit haggard in the pictures we took. Yet, the trip was worth it. At the time I still hadn't been completely diagnosed, but everything pointed to MS. In any event, I couldn't start any treatment until after I returned from Mexico and the diagnosis was confirmed.

After coming home, I went back to my routine of doctor's appointments. My neurologist asked me to try to think of any other symptoms I may have ever had. That's when it dawned on me that I should mention the trouble I had with my left leg. Up until then, I had been convinced that whatever was wrong with it was a result of my hip surgery. *"Bingo,"* the doctor said, "That's it, you have your diagnosis." Not even the results from my spinal tap were that conclusive. He then sent me to see a specialist at the Kaiser hospital in Hollywood.

After going over my story with the specialist, she told me that a traumatic event, such as a surgery can trigger a relapse of an autoimmune condition. It was all starting to make sense, except the "why?" part. When I told her about the pain I had in my right eye while I was in Mexico, she immediately set me up for an emergency IV infusion of steroids. This turned into three consecutive days of going to Kaiser with Devon and sitting for an hour while the steroids dripped into my vein. The steroids certainly did the trick for my right eye, and I'm sure other issues as well. During those three days my insurance was in the process of changing, otherwise that would have been a five day treatment. Getting new insurance meant getting new doctors, but at least now I'd know what to tell them. The doctors recommended I start the most vigorous form of treatment on the market: Tysabri.

Tysabri is a medication that is administered through an IV infusion every four weeks. It is designed for MS patients with Relapsing Remitting MS, who have not suffered enough damage that they need to use a walker or wheelchair, and patients who hopefully will prevent that type of progression. I went to my first "educational" dinner, which was funded by the company that makes Tysabri. They gave us a three course meal, freebies, and inspirational speakers. Then a doctor described what the drug did and gave all of us a scare about the possible side effects, followed by a pat on the back of reassurance that it's all worth it and necessary.

As I looked around the room, my first impression was, "I am not like these people!" Some were in wheelchairs or using canes that they leaned against the table or hooked onto their chairs. What I was really feeling, is that I did not want to become these people. I was *scared*! The representative had to tell us that this drug could kill you if you contracted a brain infection, but only if you have or are positive for PML (Progressive multifocal leukoencephalopathy). We needed to know that you must question taking Tysabri if you ever test positive for PML. Well, "This is terrible," I thought but I told myself I would do it because it was the best drug on the market.

I went in for infusions every four weeks. Sometimes I would have a panic attack after feeling symptomatic, so I'd go in a week early for my infusion. I *was* symptomatic, but again, why? I accepted that I had MS and was sick. I could barely concentrate on conversations—sometimes I felt I was staring right through someone trying to talk to me. I couldn't concentrate on their words and what was going on around me. I had chronic dry eye, and once when I got a cold I had so much pain in my face that I thought my world was crumbling. Over a period of three months I went to the ER three times—and the medical bills were piling up. In addition to Tysabri, I did two different rounds of IV steroid treatments. I also sought a second opinion from a neurologist at Keck/USC hospital. She read my MRI scans with more detail, and told me that some of the lesions caused by MS had disappeared from my MRI scans. That was exciting news!

She suggested that I have an evaluation done by a neuropsychologist. Those results were more devastating than receiving my diagnosis. That was *not* good news! I was told that I shouldn't drive far at night or long distances, that I was a poor multitasker, and that some of my functions were comparable to those of an elderly person. I cried all the way home. Thankfully I was with my husband and Devon, who were there to listen to my sob story, support me, and of course, chauffeur me.

Your	A year for change A month for change A week for change A day for change Day 22	FLog

Date:	*Sugar? FLoget about it!*	M T W TH F Sa Su

Sleep	Hours, time, quality, dreams, any A.M. symptoms? Circle a face: 😃 🙂 😐 🙁 😖

Time to eat: Solid or liquid	4am - 11am, List all ingredients, be descriptive but don't over think it.
Score:	

Symptoms:	How do you feel? See symptoms chart.

Time to eat: Solid or liquid	11am - 4pm, List all ingredients
Score:	

Symptoms:	How do you feel? See symptoms chart.

Time to eat: Solid or liquid	4pm - 8pm, List all ingredients
Score:	

Symptoms:	How do you feel? See symptoms chart.
Time to eat: Solid or liquid **Score:**	8pm - 4am, List all ingredients
Symptoms:	How do you feel? See symptoms chart.

H2O Per 8oz	Exercise, Minutes and type Anaerobic:	Minutes and type Aerobic:	Stool Analysis, time, type and the face you made
Supplements and/ or medication, other medical related logging AM: YES/NO PM: YES/NO			☺ ☺ ☻ ☹ 😖 ☺ ☺ ☻ ☹ 😖 ☺ ☺ ☻ ☹ 😖
Notes, thoughts and goals for the day ☺ ☺ ☻ ☹ 😖		Goals for tomorrow	The day's score A+ - F 0 = A+, 1-2 = A, 3-4 = A-, 5-6 = B+, 7-9 = B, 10-12 = B-,13-15 = C+ 16-18 = C, 19-21 = C-, 22-24 = D+, 25-27 = D, 28+ = F Your Grade:

Your	A year for change A month for change A week for change A day for change Day 23	**FLog**

Date:	*FLog about it!*	M T W TH F Sa Su

Sleep

Hours, time, quality, dreams, any A.M. symptoms? Circle a face:

😀 🙂 😐 🙁 😖

Time to eat: Solid or liquid

4am - 11am, List all ingredients, be descriptive but don't over think it.

Score:

Symptoms:

How do you feel? See symptoms chart.

Time to eat: Solid or liquid

11am - 4pm, List all ingredients

Score:

Symptoms:

How do you feel? See symptoms chart.

Time to eat: Solid or liquid

4pm - 8pm, List all ingredients

Score:

Symptoms:	How do you feel? See symptoms chart.
Time to eat: Solid or liquid **Score:**	8pm - 4am, List all ingredients
Symptoms:	How do you feel? See symptoms chart.

H2O Per 8oz	Exercise, Minutes and type Anaerobic:	Minutes and type Aerobic:	Stool Analysis, time, type and the face you made
Supplements and/ or medication, other medical related logging AM: YES/NO PM: YES/NO			☺ ☺ ☺ ☹ 😖 ☺ ☺ ☺ ☹ 😖 ☺ ☺ ☺ ☹ 😖
Notes, thoughts and goals for the day ☺ ☺ ☺ ☹ 😖		Goals for tomorrow	The day's score A+ - F 0 = A+, 1-2 = A, 3-4 = A-, 5-6 = B+, 7-9 = B, 10-12 = B-,13-15 = C+ 16-18 = C, 19-21 = C-, 22-24 = D+, 25-27 = D, 28+ = F Your Grade:

Your	A year for change A month for change A week for change A day for change Day 24	FLog

Date:	*If you messed up, you have hours ahead of you to choose better.*	M T W TH F Sa Su

Sleep	Hours, time, quality, dreams, any A.M. symptoms? Circle a face: ☺ ☺ ☺ ☹ 😣

Time to eat: Solid or liquid	4am - 11am, List all ingredients, be descriptive but don't over think it.
Score:	

Symptoms:	How do you feel? See symptoms chart.

Time to eat: Solid or liquid	11am - 4pm, List all ingredients
Score:	

Symptoms:	How do you feel? See symptoms chart.

Time to eat: Solid or liquid	4pm - 8pm, List all ingredients
Score:	

Symptoms:	How do you feel? See symptoms chart.
Time to eat: **Solid or** **liquid** **Score:**	8pm - 4am, List all ingredients
Symptoms:	How do you feel? See symptoms chart.

H2O Per 8oz	Exercise, Minutes and type Anaerobic:	Minutes and type Aerobic:	Stool Analysis, time, type and the face you made
Supplements and/ or medication, other medical related logging AM: YES/NO PM: YES/NO			☺ ☺ ☺ ☹ 😖 ☺ ☺ ☺ ☹ 😖 ☺ ☺ ☺ ☹ 😖
Notes, thoughts and goals for the day ☺ ☺ ☺ ☹ 😖		Goals for tomorrow	The day's score A+ - F 0 = A+, 1-2 = A, 3-4 = A-, 5-6 = B+, 7-9 = B, 10-12 = B-, 13-15 = C+ 16-18 = C, 19-21 = C-, 22-24 = D+, 25-27 = D, 28+ = F Your Grade:

Your	A year for change A month for change A week for change A day for change Day 25	FLog

Date:	*Muscle use helps regulate blood sugar and insulin levels. PUMP IT UP! (4)*	M T W TH F Sa Su

Sleep	Hours, time, quality, dreams, any A.M. symptoms? Circle a face: 😃 🙂 😐 🙁 😖

Time to eat: Solid or liquid	4am - 11am, List all ingredients, be descriptive but don't over think it.
Score:	

Symptoms:	How do you feel? See symptoms chart.

Time to eat: Solid or liquid	11am - 4pm, List all ingredients
Score:	

Symptoms:	How do you feel? See symptoms chart.

Time to eat: Solid or liquid	4pm - 8pm, List all ingredients
Score:	

Symptoms:	How do you feel? See symptoms chart.
Time to eat: **Solid or liquid**	8pm - 4am, List all ingredients
Score:	
Symptoms:	How do you feel? See symptoms chart.

H2O Per 8oz	Exercise, Minutes and type Anaerobic:	Minutes and type Aerobic:	Stool Analysis, time, type and the face you made
Supplements and/ or medication, other medical related logging AM: YES/NO			😀 🙂 😐 🙁 😣 😀 🙂 😐 🙁 😣 😀 🙂 😐 🙁 😣
PM: YES/NO			
Notes, thoughts and goals for the day 😀 🙂 😐 🙁 😣		Goals for tomorrow	The day's score A+ - F 0 = A+, 1-2 = A, 3-4 = A-, 5-6 = B+, 7-9 = B, 10-12 = B-,13-15 = C+ 16-18 = C, 19-21 = C-, 22-24 = D+, 25-27 = D, 28+ = F Your Grade:

Your	A year for change A month for change A week for change A day for change Day 26	**FLog**

Date:	***Learn to say NO! Practice makes almost perfect.***	M T W TH F Sa Su

Sleep	Hours, time, quality, dreams, any A.M. symptoms? Circle a face: 😀 ☺ 😐 ☹ 😫

Time to eat: Solid or liquid **Score:**	4am - 11am, List all ingredients, be descriptive but don't over think it.

Symptoms:	How do you feel? See symptoms chart.

Time to eat: Solid or liquid **Score:**	11am - 4pm, List all ingredients

Symptoms:	How do you feel? See symptoms chart.

Time to eat: Solid or liquid **Score:**	4pm - 8pm, List all ingredients

Symptoms:	How do you feel? See symptoms chart.
Time to eat: Solid or liquid **Score:**	8pm - 4am, List all ingredients
Symptoms:	How do you feel? See symptoms chart.

H2O Per 8oz	Exercise, Minutes and type Anaerobic:	Minutes and type Aerobic:	Stool Analysis, time, type and the face you made
Supplements and/ or medication, other medical related logging AM: YES/NO PM: YES/NO			😀 🙂 😐 🙁 😖 😀 🙂 😐 🙁 😖 😀 🙂 😐 🙁 😖
Notes, thoughts and goals for the day 😀 🙂 😐 🙁 😖		Goals for tomorrow	The day's score A+ - F 0 = A+, 1-2 = A, 3-4 = A-, 5-6 = B+, 7-9 = B, 10-12 = B-,13-15 = C+ 16-18 = C, 19-21 = C-, 22-24 = D+, 25-27 = D, 28+ = F Your Grade:

Your	A year for change A month for change A week for change A day for change Day 27	FLog

Date:	*Natural antibacterial: Berberine. Taken as a supplement can help reduce the symptoms of diabetes, high cholesterol, obesity, SIBO, lung inflammation, cancer, Alzheimer's and heart disease (5)*	M T W TH F Sa Su
Sleep	Hours, time, quality, dreams, any A.M. symptoms? Circle a face: 😀 🙂 😐 🙁 😣	
Time to eat: Solid or liquid **Score:**	4am - 11am, List all ingredients, be descriptive but don't over think it.	
Symptoms:	How do you feel? See symptoms chart.	
Time to eat: Solid or liquid **Score:**	11am - 4pm, List all ingredients	
Symptoms:	How do you feel? See symptoms chart.	
Time to eat: Solid or liquid **Score:**	4pm - 8pm, List all ingredients	

Symptoms:	How do you feel? See symptoms chart.
Time to eat: Solid or liquid **Score:**	8pm - 4am, List all ingredients
Symptoms:	How do you feel? See symptoms chart.

H2O Per 8oz	Exercise, Minutes and type Anaerobic:	Minutes and type Aerobic:	Stool Analysis, time, type and the face you made
Supplements and/ or medication, other medical related logging AM: YES/NO PM: YES/NO			🙂 🙂 😐 🙁 😖 🙂 🙂 😐 🙁 😖 🙂 🙂 😐 🙁 😖
Notes, thoughts and goals for the day 🙂 🙂 😐 🙁 😖		Goals for tomorrow	The day's score A+ - F 0 = A+, 1-2 = A, 3-4 = A-, 5-6 = B+, 7-9 = B, 10-12 = B-,13-15 = C+ 16-18 = C, 19-21 = C-, 22-24 = D+, 25-27 = D, 28+ = F Your Grade:

Your	A year for change A month for change A week for change A day for change Day 28	FLog

Date:	**_Getting FLogtigued? Get some inspiration from a colorful mix of vegetables on your plate today, to out do any Picasso!_**	M T W TH F Sa Su

Sleep	Hours, time, quality, dreams, any A.M. symptoms? Circle a face: 😃 🙂 😐 🙁 😖

Time to eat: Solid or liquid Score:	4am - 11am, List all ingredients, be descriptive but don't over think it.

Symptoms:	How do you feel? See symptoms chart.

Time to eat: Solid or liquid Score:	11am - 4pm, List all ingredients

Symptoms:	How do you feel? See symptoms chart.

Time to eat: Solid or liquid Score:	4pm - 8pm, List all ingredients

Symptoms:	How do you feel? See symptoms chart.
Time to eat: Solid or liquid **Score:**	8pm - 4am, List all ingredients
Symptoms:	How do you feel? See symptoms chart.

H2O Per 8oz	Exercise, Minutes and type Anaerobic:	Minutes and type Aerobic:	Stool Analysis, time, type and the face you made
Supplements and/ or medication, other medical related logging AM: YES/NO PM: YES/NO			😀 🙂 😐 🙁 😣 😀 🙂 😐 🙁 😣 😀 🙂 😐 🙁 😣
Notes, thoughts and goals for the day 😀 🙂 😐 🙁 😣		Goals for tomorrow	The day's score A+ - F 0 = A+, 1-2 = A, 3-4 = A-, 5-6 = B+, 7-9 = B, 10-12 = B-,13-15 = C+ 16-18 = C, 19-21 = C-, 22-24 = D+, 25-27 = D, 28+ = F Your Grade:

Cheat sheet

Water intake goal:	Exercise goal:	Supplements and/or medication:	Sleep:
Women: 91oz Men: 125oz This really does mean just plain water or a water based non-sugar based liquid like herbal tea	3-4 days a week 20-45minutes Anaerobic, aerobic (cardio) or both	Record that your took them either in the AM or PM. Record any other pertinent information. i.e. if you need to record blood pressure, ketones, blood sugar etc.	Goal 7-8 hours Keep a regular sleep/wake schedule Before sleep, do gentle stretches or meditate 5-10 minutes to fall asleep

Stool Analysis: Goal 3-4	Food law, simple list.	See Food Law pages for detailed food lists	
1 - hard to pass small lumps 2 - lumpy hard sausage like 3 - sausage like with cracks on surface 4 - like a smooth soft sausage 5 - soft blobs with clear edges 6 - mushy consistency with ragged edges 7 - liquid consistency with no solid pieces	**High risk:** Gluten Soy Corn Dairy Legumes Grains Sugar Alternative Sweetners	**Medium Risk:** Nightshades Whey Sheep's milk Food additives NSAIDs Alcohol	**Low Risk:** All eggs Nuts* Seeds* Ghee Stevia Emulsifiers/thickeners FODMAPs

Symptoms	How do you feel?		
Digestive: Diarrhea Constipation Nausea Gas Bloating Cramps Indigestion Burping Cravings Acid reflux Heartburn GERD	**Cognitive/Cerebral:** Headache Migraine Brain fog ADD/ADHD Lack of focus Fatigue Memory loss Anxiety Sleeplessness, Depression Anger Vertigo Hearing loss Vision loss Vision/blurry/spotty/pain	**Hormonal:** Heat flash Mood swing Irregular period PMS Thyroid disfunction Decreased libido Weight gain Infertility Breast tenderness Low muscle mass Heavier/lighter bleeding Back ache cramps	**Body:** Acne Hives Rash itching Sweating Joint pain Muscle ache Gout Arthritis Swelling Numbness/tingling Body/breath odor Dry eye Hair loss High blood pressure

Chapter 4

A Few Clues Are Revealed

I finally found a dermatologist willing to listen to my woes and look closely at my skin—which by now was falling apart. The other dermatologists before simply blamed my condition on washing away my skin's natural barrier repeatedly through the day as a massage therapist. They also said that it was unlikely due to food, because that was only common in children. My unspoken thought was, *"Seriously, doctor?"*

Dr. Hartman in Encino, California, was the one who finally hit the nail on the head, "This is something you're doing everyday," he told me. I thought I was super healthy, and full of confidence, I told him about all my daily supplements. He told me to stop taking all the supplements, even the whey protein in my morning juice/smoothie. I followed his advice, and not even three days later my skin was already feeling some relief. I looked at all the labels on my supplements and the common denominator was soy. Soy *had* to be the culprit! I had to clear soy from every food, drink, supplement, and even body care products that I used. I had to eventually peek at the massage cream label I used for work and Lo and behold—there was soybean oil in it. I felt like such a fool. Of course my hands and arms, especially my elbows, were going to be the most affected. I was practically swimming in the stuff up to six days a week!

This had been a rather long journey, but the best part was just beginning. Even though the journey was about to get a bit tougher, I was where I needed to be. I was no longer able to run a mile on the treadmill. High heels and I were no longer a good combination. I could walk in them for about ten minutes before I needed help because my left ankle felt like it was going to collapse. I was determined that going to nightclubs with my girls was worth it, even if they had to watch out for me. I bought many different pairs of "Going out" shoes: short heels, tall heels, fat heels, wedges, high boots, and low boots. Hardly any of them worked, but to this day I still can't let them go, even if I can't wear them. Sometimes I put on a favorite pair just to see my reflection in the mirror. Perhaps one day I'll be able to walk in them again. I do miss wearing my heels!

More than I missed the heels—I missed horses with a passion! It was time to figure out if I could still manage to ride. But I was so full of questions: could I still ride, or even want to? Would I fall? Would the horse understand my challenges? I had been an instructor, I knew these answers! Of course I could ride, of course the horse would adjust to me. Yes, I knew it would be ok. Still, my insecurities held me back for a year, until I decided to seek answers from the people at Ride On, whom I had previously worked with. I knew I could trust them, but I didn't see myself as the same person and definitely not as the same rider. It had been over two years since I last rode a horse and over four years since I had ridden on a regular basis. I wondered if I would be able to face and conquer the changes in my body. Thanks to the kindness of the people at Ride On, I finally got back on a horse—although now as a student. Ride On was incredibly kind to not charge me for these first few lessons that, for me, were experimental at best.

Even though I had plenty of experience riding and as an instructor, I still didn't know what to expect of this turn as a student. I was faced with many doubts, and the control I used to have, was now a thing of the past. Could I handle an instructor telling me how to do simple things? Nevertheless, I was extremely thankful that I got to try. At first the horse only walked and I had my movements analyzed. I was analyzing my body as well. My control was gone, I felt vulnerable, and others could see my limitations and struggles. I cried in the car for twenty minutes after I finished my first lesson.

How do you give up the reins? Fate had led me to a place beyond my control and comfort zone. It's easy to look at where you want to go and who you want to be when you feel in control of your path. Eventually you have to go down one of two paths, uncertain of what you will encounter. I always had a feeling that I would be challenged with something very dear to me—a person, a thing—just not *me*! Destiny and God's plan can play tricks on us. Hindsight is 20/20. You never know how the challenges happening in your life now may be preparing you for your future.

I never thought I would be forced to face something I didn't want, or something I couldn't change. I can't change that I was diagnosed with Multiple Sclerosis. I can't change that my body made a mistake and changed in a way I didn't want. I can't change that the left side of my body doesn't work like it used to. I *can* decide how I'll feel, and which path I'll take. Follow your dreams and talents because they have been chosen especially for you so that you can change the lives of others.

I enjoy riding now more than ever. I have gone from a basic walk lesson where I didn't touch the reins, to more advanced independent walk, trot and canter lessons. Dressage lessons are tough, but they challenge both sides of my brain and body and have long lasting effects which are helping to improve my everyday functions. I may have a bad limp after I dismount, constantly lose my left stirrup, and the reins slip through my fingers all the time, but those problems continue to improve little by little with all the help of my lifestyle changes and my positive attitude.

Today horses are my therapy. In the past horses were a recreational activity and a job that I could do in any weather, all day, five days a week. Although my therapeutic riding instructor and frequent recreational riding days are over, my story in the saddle continues.

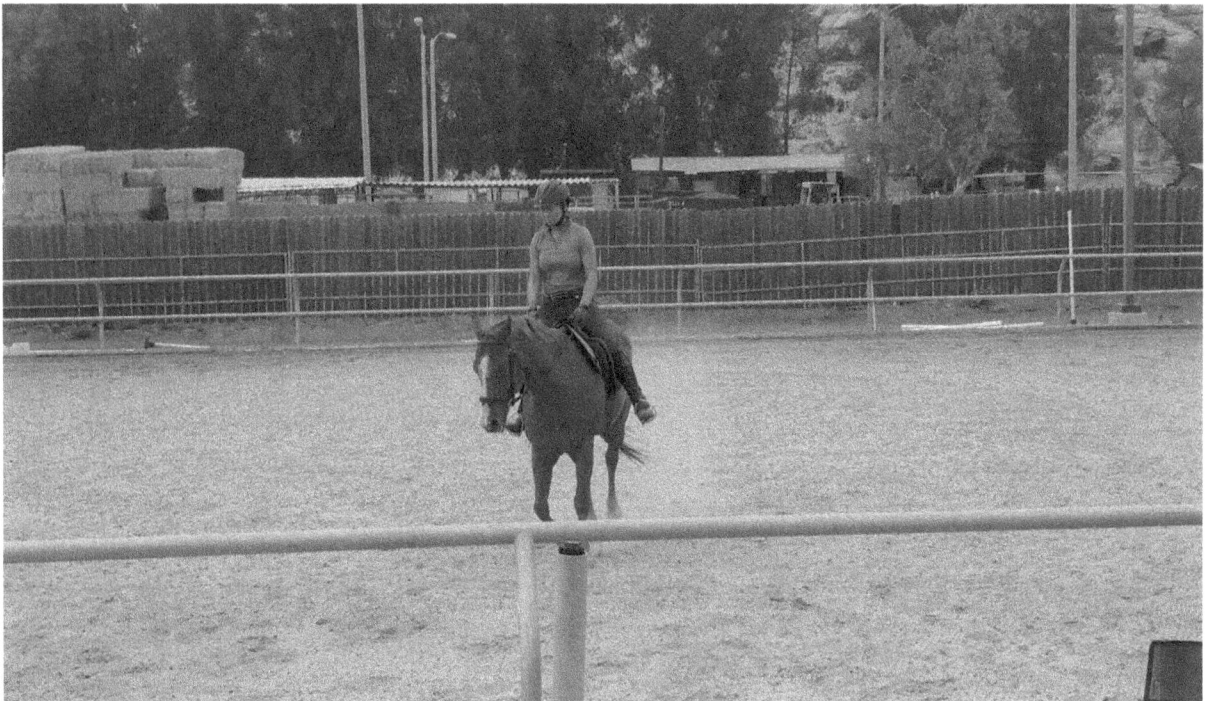

Your	A year for change A month for change A week for change A day for change Day 29	FLog

Date:	*Have you talked to a FLogMentor today?* M T W TH F Sa Su

Sleep	Hours, time, quality, dreams, any A.M. symptoms? Circle a face: 😛 ☺ 😐 ☹ 😖

Time to eat: Solid or liquid	4am - 11am, List all ingredients, be descriptive but don't over think it.
Score:	

Symptoms:	How do you feel? See symptoms chart.

Time to eat: Solid or liquid	11am - 4pm, List all ingredients
Score:	

Symptoms:	How do you feel? See symptoms chart.

Time to eat: Solid or liquid	4pm - 8pm, List all ingredients
Score:	

Symptoms:	How do you feel? See symptoms chart.
Time to eat: Solid or liquid **Score:**	8pm - 4am, List all ingredients
Symptoms:	How do you feel? See symptoms chart.

H2O Per 8oz	Exercise, Minutes and type Anaerobic:	Minutes and type Aerobic:	Stool Analysis, time, type and the face you made
Supplements and/ or medication, other medical related logging AM: YES/NO PM: YES/NO			🙂 🙂 😐 🙁 😣 🙂 🙂 😐 🙁 😣 🙂 🙂 😐 🙁 😣
Notes, thoughts and goals for the day 🙂 🙂 😐 🙁 😣		Goals for tomorrow	The day's score A+ - F 0 = A+, 1-2 = A, 3-4 = A-, 5-6 = B+, 7-9 = B, 10-12 = B-,13-15 = C+ 16-18 = C, 19-21 = C-, 22-24 = D+, 25-27 = D, 28+ = F Your Grade:

Your	A year for change A month for change A week for change A day for change Day 30	**FLog**

Date:	***Choose to FLog***	M T W TH F Sa Su
Sleep	Hours, time, quality, dreams, any A.M. symptoms? Circle a face: 😃 🙂 😐 🙁 😖	
Time to eat: **Solid or** **liquid** **Score:**	4am - 11am, List all ingredients, be descriptive but don't over think it.	
Symptoms:	How do you feel? See symptoms chart.	
Time to eat: **Solid or** **liquid** **Score:**	11am - 4pm, List all ingredients	
Symptoms:	How do you feel? See symptoms chart.	
Time to eat: **Solid or** **liquid** **Score:**	4pm - 8pm, List all ingredients	

Symptoms:	How do you feel? See symptoms chart.
Time to eat: Solid or liquid	8pm - 4am, List all ingredients
Score:	
Symptoms:	How do you feel? See symptoms chart.

H2O Per 8oz	Exercise, Minutes and type Anaerobic:	Minutes and type Aerobic:	Stool Analysis, time, type and the face you made
Supplements and/ or medication, other medical related logging AM: YES/NO PM: YES/NO			🙂 🙂 😐 🙁 😖 🙂 🙂 😐 🙁 😖 🙂 🙂 😐 🙁 😖
Notes, thoughts and goals for the day 🙂 🙂 😐 🙁 😖		Goals for tomorrow	The day's score A+ - F 0 = A+, 1-2 = A, 3-4 = A-, 5-6 = B+, 7-9 = B, 10-12 = B-,13-15 = C+ 16-18 = C, 19-21 = C-, 22-24 = D+, 25-27 = D, 28+ = F Your Grade:

Chapter 5

Finding the Answers to My "Why?"

I was eventually able to help support myself and my husband by running my massage business out of a great local gym. By the age of 33 I had built my reputation and increased my clientele to the point where I no longer needed to juggle three jobs. I needed something for myself, I had seen other "support" groups and they were mostly full of people who complained and felt sorry for themselves. I didn't want to be around that because I was already kind of doing that to myself. Instead, I was trying to create a "MeetUp" group for people with MS like me. I had faith that if I could lift up others, then they would also lift up me. My first meeting was attended by only one person—but it was meant to be.

The first member in my group walked in with an incredible story of bravery. I thought we were a match made in heaven. It turned out we actually attended the same church, though we had not met because it is one of the biggest churches in Los Angeles: Shepherd of the Hills, in Porter Ranch. By the second meeting we started talking about diet, and determined we actually had a similar vegetarian diet. She told me about a free online seminar hosted by Dr. Amy Myers, called the Autoimmune Summit. We both signed up and committed ourselves to listening to every single talk for seven days straight. I was hooked from the first interview. The Summit's speakers told a completely new story on health. They described what a leaky gut is, what foods contribute to it and why. There's that word again, "Why". That was the question no one in my health journey had been able to solve so far. That week changed my outlook on why the right fats are important, why animal fats are more crucial to some individuals than others, and *why* soy is *bad*!

I finally figured out why the plaques on my arms would literally weep clear fluid if I ate a flour tortilla. *Ding, ding, ding*: Gluten plus soy was a double shot of inflammation! By the time the online summit was over and I had listened to the healing testimonies of others, I bought Dr. Amy Myers' book, started the elimination AIP (autoimmune protocol) diet, and I also signed up for the next summit by Dr. Josh Axe, and the next summit by Donna Gates, and so on. I absorbed as much information as possible and took a lot of notes so that the next time I got together with my new "MeetUp" friend we could go over our new food protocol. This protocol evolved into what is now the Food Law in The FLog. After doing Dr. Myers' Autoimmune Protocol elimination diet, for eight weeks, I went from 160 pounds to 142 pounds. This was my lightest weight ever as an adult. I was sold on following the AIP guidelines, not only because my jean size dropped but because I was beginning to feel myself again: confident and ready to spread the word about what I was changing in my life.

God had sent me a person who brought great change. We tried to gather more people into our group but it never took off. It turned out I only really needed to meet one person. Much love to you Lexie! God works in mysterious ways. Feeling more stable with my health was huge. Carrying on conversations with a smile on my face felt amazing! I even felt confident enough to drive myself to my parent's house, two hours away. I managed to make the drive, but I realized that I wasn't quite ready for that challenge. It was incredible how the neuropsychologist's analysis affected my confidence and ability. I didn't know whether to completely believe the neuropsychology evaluation, if my brain had just not been ready, or if I simply did not have the confidence. Two years after my first attempt, I successfully tried the drive again. That was a win that meant it was possible to improve.

Over the next few months, the thought started bouncing around in my head, "Do I still need Tysabri?" It was a scary thought but also one that challenged my faith. The eight week elimination process had been very successful in stifling the inflammation in my body, but it was just the start.

I started shopping at health food stores, which opened up a pandora's box of tasty foods that seemed safe for me ingredient-wise. I tried a lot of these foods and I gained back about five pounds. Two ingredients I was never going to reintroduce to my sensitive GI tract were gluten and soy, which are my body's kryptonite ingredients. Old habits die hard, so I reduced my occasional fast food intake to french fries and cheesy bean cups. Of course, I had to make sure they weren't made with soybean oil! I had this soy ingredient elimination rule down to the T. Reintroducing meat and eggs was a slow process as my diet changed. It had been over six years since I last had them and I was pretty convinced that the texture would make me gag. My options were limited, to say the least, and I was still baby-stepping my way through finding foods I could eat. Once I was a 'meat eater' again, a certain fast food chain introduced their 'natural burger'. I ordered it lettuce wrapped when I was 'desperate' for food, short on time, or when there were no other options available. Over time, that burger started to taste flavorless. The cheese and beans wrecked my stomach, and corn was starting to give me a rash. It was time to say goodbye to more bad habits.

It didn't take my taste buds long to realize organic animal protein was really delicious, *especially* bacon. I was referred to very good quality organic meat companies, which made that transition easier because clean meat tastes better. Some of those companies are listed on the resource pages of The FLog. After this change in diet, my body started to build muscle like never before. Those skinny jeans didn't fit over my butt again, although for a good reason: I gained ten pounds of muscle.

My food sensitivities started to become more and more obvious. Corn and nuts were causing my arms to itch and I'd get hives around my elbows whenever I ate them. Too much bad sugar gave me brain fog, garlic and chocolate gave me the farts, and any type of grain or legume made me bloated. Some nights an arm would go numb and I'd awake from a dead sleep in excruciating pain as it slowly regained feeling. As you read in previous chapters, this used to happen regularly: at least once or twice a week. I no longer accepted these symptoms as normal. As my diet got cleaner and less inflammatory, I became hyper aware of how my body reacted to certain foods or ingredients. I learned to listen to my body, record how it felt, and began connecting the dots between what I consumed and my body's reactions. Some things were harder to figure out, but I kept narrowing it down and educating myself.

That was when I started logging my food in a little daily journal I had. I wrote down what I ate and how I felt anytime after. Then I starting adding in my bowel movements and sleep. Then came exercise routines and so on. I needed to log because I would easily forget what I had eaten. If I had not recorded it, it was difficult to connect the dots between food and symptoms. I was also learning what all my symptoms actually were. Learning to read labels was challenging and narrowing down what food chemicals or emulsifiers affected me was like learning a whole new science.

The FLog took about two years to create just by learning to do it for myself and another year to figure out a user friendly way for others to implement it. Which is in no way easy to learn how to do. You will eventually catch onto the routine. You're taking a front row class into figuring out your own body. The FLog is not designed for you to do only for a little while. There will always be a new product at the grocery store which appears to be within your food protocol—and you're going to try it. There will be times when you're at a restaurant or bar and might want to try something on the menu. Your diet will never stay exactly the same. It will change because your body will change. The FLog will help you record every successful day, every day you tried something new, and those days in which you gave in to temptation and fell off the boat. You'll notice what the repercussions may be for that ingredient.

Eventually, the tremor in my left arm began to slowly improve and tasks like chopping vegetables became a little easier. A huge sign of improvement was being able to lift my arm in church to give God some praise. When the tremor first started, my husband would help me lift my arm at church by holding it anchored in his own arm. This was very sweet of him, but I wanted to do it on my own. This gave me another reason to keep my faith strong and stay on the right food path. I was able to tap my left foot to the music with a little more rhythm! I still keep my own healing prayer attached to the inside of my front door at home. I recorded that prayer onto my phone so I can listen to myself speak the words out loud, "God is my healer." I was, and still am, determined to stay faithful and remind myself that all is possible through God.

Excerpt from my healing prayer, written by Susanna Nicole:

I give no place to sickness or pain because God sent his word and healed me. I thank you for giving me abundant life, and I receive that life through your word and it flows through every organ in my body bringing health and healing.

Therefore, I refuse to allow MS to dominate my body, the life of God flows within me bringing healing to the insulating covers of my nerve cells in my brain and spinal cord. My nervous system will not be disrupted. Instead it communicates perfectly to every organ, muscle and tissue in my body. I command inflammation plaques and lesions to go because Jesus bore the curse for me. I declare I am healed and refuse to allow MS to operate in my body, and I declare that my strength and health are restored. Thank you Lord, that you have blessed my food my water and have taken sickness away from me. I will fulfill the number of my days in health and prosperity, Amen.

I did not skip this prayer even during my lowest and sickest days. I will continue to say it, because in ten years I will look back and see how much I have accomplished, achieved and healed. I also pray that I will reach and help many others, and that they too will reach people in their lives who need a healthier lifestyle.

Chapter 6

Revelations

I have told my story to people in my circle of trust and to those whom I felt I could help. They often told me that I should write a book, but I had doubts as to whether I could put my thoughts on paper. I am *not a* writer! I also did not think anyone would take the time to read it. This book is not only about helping you change your life, but also about how I changed my life and overcame the challenges of autoimmunity. In reflection, autoimmune symptoms were present throughout most of my life. When you don't know that you have autoimmunity, you end up on a long journey of finding out what is wrong and how to address it. Life is an unpredictable and challenging experience. It can be calm seas or a tidal wave. Sometimes I feel that autoimmunity is waiting to devour me, but I remind myself, that I am standing on it; it is not standing on me or in my way. Multiple sclerosis has left physical scars in and on my body. Some are healing or even disappeared, while others are still lingering. Some may never go away, but as long as I keep healing, I know that *I am* succeeding.

It took six months to find the answer to that question that had been bouncing around in my head, "Do I still need Tysabri, or could I do this with diet and faith alone?" I knew the differences in my body were real and I also knew that if I needed medication it would be there for me to fall back on. But, I had to make this decision with 100% confidence. I was going to do this and trust it, or not do it at all. I couldn't think about the medication, only my choices of food. I also knew that I would be making this decision without my doctor's support. I had to go in to that doctor's office with my head held high and tell her I had decided to go off medication. Predictably, she responded by asking why I wanted to stop, since it seemed to be helping and I wasn't having any obvious negative effects from it. She was right, at least as far as I could tell. Still, I needed to know how I'd feel without it.

My neurologist and I agreed that I could always go back on the drug if I needed it. I'm positive she expected me to go back on Tysabri sooner or later. How many patients take their health into their own hands using diet? Apparently not enough to give conventional medicine a different reputation. I made my decision being fully confident that I'd never go back on medication. I am not in any way advocating that you stop taking any medication that has been prescribed by a doctor, but I do believe that you should consider your options. Analyze your situation—perhaps you can reduce your need for medication and supplements through lifestyle and diet changes. You may never be able to go off medication completely, but it may be possible to go on lower doses or less extreme immunosuppressants.

My last Tysabri infusion was October 2015, almost three years ago as I am writing this story. I have never felt progressive or symptomatic during that time. I know most of the symptoms I suffered most of my life were all due to inflammation from what I put in my body, and how my genes respond to these factors.

Even as my health improved, my intuition told me that my body was a little burdened by the paleo-type diet I had followed for over two years. I was not having regular bowel movements. I had never in my life experienced the kind of constipation that caused me to pass out before, but it happened. I had never needed a suppository before, but I had to use them a few times during this uncomfortable time period. The suppositories did what they are intended to do, but my digestive system would still be reeling days later. Why was I constipated every few weeks?

I thought perhaps it was the "gluten free" or "grain free" breads that were causing me digestive problems. I figured the doughy consistency was acting like wet concrete in my intestines. I had to make some changes. I felt frustrated and thought about going vegetarian or pescatarian again because even my "good" diet was holding me back. I had some belly fat that hadn't been there before in my pescatarian days. *WTFLog?* Why was I gaining fat around my midsection and feeling a little run down?

It turned out that the coconut flour, arrowroot starch, and grain free breads were not the main cause of my problems. I had to re-evaluate their presence in my diet, because they still had ingredients I shouldn't have been eating. Just because something says, "gluten free" or it's a trendy product that's being hyped as the next miracle food, it doesn't mean it is actually good for your particular body.

You might be as surprised to find out that it was the amount of animal protein I was consuming, which really wasn't that excessive. I challenged myself to go from having animal protein every one to two meals a day, to one to two days a week. This did not include the bone broth; I was still allowing myself the protein and fat from broths three or more days a week.

One week after starting this new regime, I was pooping one, two and even three times a day! I thought, *"Where the poo was all this coming from?"* All that animal protein in my diet was stopping my motility (movement in the intestines). My body felt so much relief after I cut down my animal protein. This may not be the best plan for you, but your particular lifestyle may not need animal protein everyday. Even some athletes perform best as vegans. In fact, you may know some of those athletes or you may be one yourself. We are all different, so be flexible with your diet. You may think the things you eat are the best, but there may be something better for you out there.

Eventually I started to take a little of everything I had learned and created my body's unique food protocol. I didn't need to be put in only one category of eaters. I can be a vegan for a day or even a week; I can eat meat sparingly because my body doesn't seem to need it every day. It does need healthy fats and nutrients from animals, so I make my own bone broths. I've learned to eat foods of the earth that work for me. I'm normally tempted to try new foods that don't necessarily give me the best reactions, but I learn from my mistakes and get smarter everyday about keeping my body happy and healthy. Food *can* be medicine!

As a result of my new diet, I did lose some of the belly fat I mentioned before. Fasting has also played a big role in maintaining muscle mass while losing fat. It's interesting how one's body changes. In the past I could lose fat around my middle section first and then on my legs, but now it's the opposite. My jeans fit over my butt once again and the scale hadn't changed at 152 pounds. I'm not a scientist and admittedly I don't understand it all, but I'll keep playing around with my body chemistry as long as I keep seeing improvements.

Since most people tend to eat the same things on a regular basis, it's really not too hard to start narrowing down the food or ingredients that affect you negatively. It's all in the details, like chemicals, emulsifiers, preservatives, or "natural" ingredients (whatever the heck those are) that you don't usually realize are in the foods you eat. There are days where I eat super clean, then go out with friends and drink the wrong kind of alcohol. I typically look up which alcoholic drinks are gluten free or which wines are organic. Just like I do with my food, I must research these things too. I know what you're thinking, "Why not just give up drinking alcohol at social events or altogether?" Well, that's part of my struggle. I enjoy a nice cocktail every now and then. What is your struggle? Whatever it is, you will see that it gets easier as you start to see how your body deals with inflammation and how much better you feel without an inflamed body and brain. Remember, feeling amazing is addictive!

I struggled with feelings of depression when I was first diagnosed. Having resources and a support system is very important. My health insurance at the time had a call center that actually checked up on me. I was even asked if I had feelings of suicide or extreme depression. At one point I answered yes, which was very hard for me to admit. They were quick to put me in contact with a program that called me once a week, provided cognitive behavior lessons over the phone, and provided worksheets to understand my feelings and how to express myself. I cried during some of those phone calls and released a lot of the emotions I couldn't release with anyone else. This program helped me more than I thought was possible. On their recommendation, I tried another therapist but I found I no longer needed it. It's hard to feel better, put on a brave face, and face the world, but you have to try. Pray on it, cry it out, or share your story with someone who can give you the right tools to understand yourself. Meditate on peacefulness because you can get through anything.

Wanting to feel better means acting like you feel better, having a positive attitude and pushing yourself to wellness. In order to be well, *you have to believe in yourself,* and you have to show people that you're doing well.

My early symptoms fell into many categories of autoimmune disease. I could have been diagnosed with restless leg syndrome, fibromyalgia or any number of other autoimmune diseases. The diagnosis came down to identifying symptoms, medical scans, blood work, and my doctors' knowledge. I encourage you to believe in my story and the story of so many others who have healed themselves through food. Food as medicine is real. You can use it alone or in conjunction with necessary medication. It's ok to question science because that's what science is—trial and error. There's a little scientist in all of us.

It took four years to slowly stop waking up with muscle spasms or with numb arms followed by excruciating pain. When that happens, it's because I ate or drank an inflammatory substance. I can almost always find the pattern between certain foods and symptoms. In the past, solutions like foam rolling or stretching helped my muscles feel a little better but did not address what was causing the symptom of muscle spasm. If you get to the root of the problem, you'll stop beating your head against a wall trying to figure out why you don't feel good.

In addition to my non-inflammatory diet, I use chemical free household cleaners and chemical free body products as much as possible. I filter my water and drink a lot of it and I make my own toothpaste and deodorant. I diffuse essential oils and turn on my salt lamp. I buy locally sourced or organic fruits and vegetables and source meats only from humane farmers. I finally feel that I have found a great way to stay healthy and keep my immune system working well. My skin now rarely itches. "FLogging" has kept me accountable, so that my reactions to certain low risks foods are far from severe. I still have more weight to lose and more muscle to gain. I am *very* thankful that now those are my main goals instead of worrying about coping with multiple sclerosis symptoms, wheelchairs, or the fact that the tremor in my left arm has been quite the challenge when typing this book.

I hope that my story serves as an illustration that everything that happens in life is leading you somewhere. Through the grace of God I am still going strong and I don't ignore my body. You should observe your health carefully. Care with special love for those who come into your life. Listen to your doctor, but you also need to find your own special way of taking care of yourself. I owe my new found abilities to the lifestyle and dietary changes I have made through my journey, and these changes have helped my body heal and regain some function.

I thank God for my path and ask for the courage to continue living my story. As I finish writing the last chapter, I look forward to more years to prove I can be well and better. I will *pray* to God to keep me faithful and strong because I need His help. My neurologist never followed up with me since I stopped the Tysabri treatments. I am doing better than ever and will send her a copy of this book with the hope that more patients will take control of their health and/or diagnosis <u>with</u> their doctor alongside them.

WHAT'S YOUR STORY?

A letter from the Author

Congratulations, you have <u>finished</u> 30 days!

First of all you are number one in your FLog! You have taken steps and made conscious effort to succeed every day at making your body function optimally. I hope you have seen how your whole self responds to good fuel and a healthy routine. I pray you pass on the good news to people you know. Your family is first on that list. Young and old, you should want all people to live long and well. I encourage you to continue on your journey to wellness and take as many people with you on that path. Working as a team and in numbers greater than one, is always to our advantage! Thank yourself now for your *next* 30 days of FLogging! I create my own additional log pages so I can continue FLogging daily. Trouble starts to happen when I don't hold myself accountable.

AngelaLanderosHeals.wordpress.com
to stay connected
and updated on new happenings

Share the good news and be well. My sincere thanks for taking steps every day to be better.

God bless,

Angela M. Landeros
HAVE, F.A.I.T.H. = Fighting Auto Immunity Through Health

Philippians 4:13
> *I can do all things through Christ who strengthens me.*

Resources

Below is a list of scientists, naturopathic doctors and wellness entrepreneurs. You can buy their books, sign up for newsletters, and listen to free summits designed to teach you why you should eat a non-inflammatory diet. Feeling your best is contagious and you'll want to spread it around creating a ripple effect.

Dr. Amy Myers,
The Myers Way
https://www.amymyersmd.com

Dr. Josh Axe,
Eat Dirt
https://draxe.com

Dr. David Perlmutter,
Brain Maker
Grain Brain
https://www.drperlmutter.com

Dr. Eric Zalinksy,
The Healing Power of Essential Oils
https://drericz.com

Dr. Terry Wahls
Wahls Protocol
https://terrywahls.com

Dr. Mark Hyman,
Broken Brain
http://drhyman.com

Dr. Natasha Campbell-McBride,
Gut and Psychology Syndrome
http://www.gapsdiet.com/home.html

Donna Gates,
The Body Ecology Diet
https://bodyecology.com

Dr. Datis Kharrazian,
Why Isn't My Brain Working?
Why Do I Still Have Thyroid Symptoms?
https://drknews.com

Dr. Peter J. D'Adamo,
Eat Right For Your Type
Change Your Genetic Destiny
http://www.dadamo.com

Dave Asprey,
Head Strong
Creator of the bulletproof diet
https://blog.bulletproof.com

Dr. Anna Cabeca,
Keto - Alkaline Diet
Urine test strips for alkalinity and ketones
https://drannacabeca.com

Dr. Michael J. Campbell, DC.
Chiropractic Care, Sports Injury
https://www.mywoodlandhillschiropractor.com
20971 Burbank Blvd.
Woodland Hills, Ca. 91367

Go to healthtalks.com to sign up for free online summits and hear hundreds of like minded people motivated to helping anyone understand the importance of lifestyle transformation for healing the body and mind.

http://healthtalksonline.com

Where to Find Foods, Supplements, and More

Stress Management

Try hypnotherapy for stress management, meditation to engage your parasympathetic nervous system, and exercise to relieve tension and help sweat out the toxins. Here are my favorite references for a healthy mind:
- Surf City's hypnotherapy applications on your electronic devices: https://surfcityapps.com
- Meditation and yoga with Regina Queen: http://www.intheflowwellness.com
- Fitness Blender on YouTube and the web for Pilates, HIIT workouts, interval training for low and high impact and both beginners and advanced: https://www.fitnessblender.com
- Yoga and stretching on YouTube for body balance and relaxation: https://www.youtube.com/watch?v=1fztE4mK7C0

Mobility Conditioning (MobCon), foam rolling, and ball rolling with my videos on YouTube for self-massage, tissue release, and detoxification: https://www.youtube.com/c/AngelaLPTBW

US Wellness Meats

"It turns out that what's good for animals and the planet is also good for you. Our meat is tender and tasty, but it doesn't have all the excess fat of animals fed with grain in confinement. It's full of nutrients that can only come from a fully grass-fed diet—omega-3 fatty acids, vitamin A, vitamin E, and CLA—and free of all the pesticides, hormones, and antibiotics that are found in grain-fed beef. *More than just meat products too!*"

https://grasslandbeef.com

Dragon Herbs

"Dragon Herbs is a provider of health promoting herbs and complimentary services, including education and educational materials.We at Dragon Herbs know that radiant health is the result of good living and a healthy lifestyle. As a team, we are dedicated to aiding and guiding you on your path to radiant health, and to building a better world as a result. With our tonic bar, complimentary herbal consultations, and over 1000 herbal formulations made from the finest quality herbs in the world, we are sure that we can be your principal wellness center, serving the many needs you may have in order to achieve radiant health." http://www.dragonherbs.com/aboutus.asp

Safe Catch Tuna

"Our sustainability policy focuses on the entire ecosystem, meaning we look at the health of the oceans in conjunction with the health of the life it supports. We have chosen our catch methods very carefully with a great deal of support from the Monterey Bay Aquarium Seafood Watch Program. All seafood we use must first meet high standards of quality and the sustainability criteria prior to Safe Catch testing to our strict mercury standard, published on every package. If it doesn't meet our published mercury standard, we don't purchase it. We are the only seafood brand with the technology to test every single fish and we are the only brand that does." https://safecatch.com/sustainability-policy/

Vital Choice Seafood and Steaks: *(Fantastic choice for high quality fish oil supplements)*

"Vital Choice seafood is processed and flash-frozen hours within hours of harvest, preserving the fresh-caught flavor, appearance, texture, and nutritional quality of our premium quality fish and shellfish. The "fresh" fish in most markets is rarely in the ideal condition that label implies. And while many supermarkets sell previously frozen fish, it may not have been frozen quickly post-harvest, and typically languishes, thawed, in a display case for hours or days, exposed to air and light…conditions that foster bacterial growth and render delicate omega-3s rancid very quickly." https://www.vital-choice.com

Supplements:

"PureFormulas is a leader in the online health and supplement space. We specialize in offering our customers GMP certified quality products, including nutritional supplements and organic foods, as well as beauty, sports nutrition, and pet products." https://www.pureformulas.com/brand/pure-encapsulations.html?CAWELAID=1091091897&CAPCID=212586952972&-

cadevice=c&agid=1467285176&catci=kwd-801175586&gclid=EAIaIQobChMI0JHM4o_
-2AIVEf5kCh0GqALmEAAYASAAEgLctvD_BwE#

Biological Dentistry

Biological dentistry is concerned with the whole-body effects of all dental materials, techniques, and procedures. It is fluoride-free, mercury-free, and mercury-safe. Individualized testing for bio-compatibility of dental materials is a must. Biological dentistry insists that all clinical practice be designed of components that sustain life or improve the patient's quality of life, for the word "biological" refers to life. https://iabdm.org

What is functional Medicine?

Functional medicine is a systems biology–based approach that focuses on identifying and addressing the root cause of disease. Each symptom or differential diagnosis may be one of many contributing to an individual's illness. By addressing root cause rather than symptoms, practitioners become oriented to identifying the complexity of disease. They may find one condition has many different causes. Likewise, one cause may result in many different conditions. As a result, functional medicine treatment targets the specific manifestations of disease in each individual.

Find a practitioner, https://www.ifm.org/find-a-practitioner/

Daily FLog Footnotes

[1] Wikipedia. Cruciferous Vegetables. Retrieved from https://en.wikipedia.org/wiki/Cruciferous_vegetables
[2] (Feb 2018). Article: Methane emissions from cattle are 11% higher than estimated. The Guardian. Retrieved from https://www.theguardian.com/environment/2017/sep/29/methane-emissions-cattle-11-percent-higher-than-estimated
[3] Selhub, E. MD. (APRIL 05, 2018). Nutritional psychiatry: Your brain on food. Retrieved from https://www.health.harvard.edu/blog/nutritional-psychiatry-your-brain-on-food-201511168626
[4] Upham, B. (April 6, 2018). Study Reveals Potential Mechanism in Strength Training That Can Help Reduce Insulin Resistance. Retrieved from https://www.everydayhealth.com/type-2-diabetes/treatment/mechanism-strength-training-can-help-reduce-insulin-resistance/
[5] Dr. Axe, J. Article: Berberine. Retrieved from https://draxe.com/berberine/

Scripture noted:

1 Cor. 15:44 It is sown a natural body, it is raised a spiritual body. If there is a natural body, there is also a spiritual body

Philippians 4:13 I can do all things through Christ who strengthens me.

Endnotes

1 Slazenger, S, (July 29, 2015). Inflammatory Symptoms, Immune System and Food Intolerance: One cause – Many Symptoms. Retrieved from https://cellsciencesystems.com/education/research/inflammatory-symptoms-immune-system-and-food-intolerance-one-cause-many-symptoms/

2 (December 2017). The National Institute of Diabetes and Digestive and Kidney Diseases. Retrieved from https://www.niddk.nih.gov/health-information/digestive-diseases/digestive-system-how-it-works and Dr. Axe, J. How your digestive system works. Retrieved from https://draxe.com/how-your-digestive-system-works/

3 Brown, M. PhD, RD (UK) (November 12, 2017). Does Sugar Cause Inflammation in the Body? Retrieved from https://www.healthline.com/nutrition/sugar-and-inflammation#section1 and Dr. Osbourne, P. Artificial Sweeteners and Toxic Side Effects. Retrieved from https://drpeterosborne.com/artificial-sweeteners-toxic-side-effects/

4 Dr. Myers, A. (April 10, 2013). The Dangers of Dairy. Retrieved from https://www.mindbodygreen.com/0-8646/the-dangers-of-dairy.html

5 Dr. Ede, G. Grains Beans nuts and seeds. Retrieved from http://www.diagnosisdiet.com/food/grains-beans-nuts-and-seeds/

6 Joseph, M. MSc. (January 13, 2017). 11 Harmful Food Additives Hiding in Processed Food. Retrieved from https://www.nutritionadvance.com/harmful-food-additives-processed-food/ and Wikipedia, List of Food Additives. Retrieved from https://en.wikipedia.org/wiki/List_of_food_additives and Ghose, T. (February 25, 2015). Food Additives Linked to Weight Gain, Inflammation. Retrieved from https://www.livescience.com/49949-food-additives-cause-inflammation.html

7 NDTV Food (February 26, 2015). The Food Additive That Could Cause Metabolic Syndrome. Retrieved from https://food.ndtv.com/health/the-food-additive-that-could-cause-metabolic-syndrome-742660

8 Article: All About Nightshades. Paleo Leap. Retrieved from https://paleoleap.com/nightshades/

9 Virgin, J.CNS, CHFS. (September 15, 2013) Are Eggs Really Nature's Perfect Food? Retrieved from https://www.huffingtonpost.com/jj-virgin/eggs-healthy_b_3595128.html and Wikipedia, Retrieved from https://en.wikipedia.org/wiki/Egg_allergy

10 Dr. Axe, J. The Dangers of NSAIDs. Retrieved from https://draxe.com/dangers-of-nsaids/

11 Administrator of Dr. KNews. (December 27, 2017). Omega-3 fats necessary to dampen inflammation and autoimmunity. Retrieved from https://drknews.com/omega-3-fats-necessary-dampen-inflammation-autoimmunity/

12 (April 10, 2018). How Much Water Should I Drink? Retrieved from www.bodybuilding.com

13 Davis, K. (February 28, 2018). 50 Shades Of Yellow: What Color Should Your Pee Be? Retrieved from https://www.bodybuilding.com/content/50-shades-of-yellow-what-color-should-your-pee-be.html

14 Yaneff, J. CNP. (February 1, 2018). Why Is My Urine Oily? Common Causes. Retrieved from https://www.doctorshealthpress.com/bladder-articles/oily-urine-common-causes/

15 Ellis, G (March 10, 2011). Electronic Urban Repot. Retrieved from http://archive.eurweb.com/2011/03/strategies-for-well-being-bowel-movements-sinkers-or-floaters/

16 Tresca, A. (June 18, 2018). What Are the Causes of Black Stool? Retrieved from https://www.verywellhealth.com/causes-of-black-stool-1941711

17 Bolen, B. PhD (November 03, 2017). Why You Might See Blood in Your Stool. Retrieved from https://www.verywellhealth.com/blood-in-stools-1945265

18 A.D.A.M. (April 20, 2016). Stress, Penn State Hershey. Retrieved from http://pennstatehershey.adam.com/content.aspx?productId=10&pid=10&gid=000031

19 Sargis, R. MD, PhD (April 8, 2015). An Overview of the Adrenal Glands, Beyond Fight or Flight. Retrieved from https://www.endocrineweb.com/endocrinology/overview-adrenal-glands

20 Dr. Axe, J. 7 Benefits of Fasting + the Best Types of Fasting. Retrieved from https://draxe.com/benefits-fasting/

21 Gundry, S. (July 29, 2017). Labels that lie: 5 Food Labels Meant to Fool Us. Retrieved from https://www.elephantjournal.com/2017/07/labels-that-lie-5-food-labels-meant-to-fool-us/ and Bailin, D. & Goldman, G. & Phartiyal, P. (June

2014). Sugar-Coating Science: How the Food Industry Misleads Consumers on Sugar (2014). Retrieved from https://www.ucsusa.org/center-for-science-and-democracy/sugar-coating-science.html#.WvdkyS-ZNAY

22 Heritage Integrative Healthcare. Article: The Importance of Chewing Your Food. Retrieved from http://heritageihc.com/blog/chewing-your-food/

23 Shaw, H. (March 24, 2018). Before You Buy Fish, Check for Mercury Levels. Retrieved from https://www.thespruceeats.com/check-fish-for-mercury-before-buying-1300629

24 2018 Article, NSAID's List. Retrieved from http://www.nsaidslist.com

25 2018 Article, NSAID's List. Retrieved from http://www.nsaidslist.com

26 Article: What are FODMAPs. Retrieved from http://fodmapfriendly.com/what-are-fodmaps/ and Wikipedia, FODMAP's. Retrieved from https://en.wikipedia.org/wiki/FODMAP

27 (November 20, 2017). Article: The Low FODMAP Diet Approach: Measuring FODMAPs in Foods Retrieved from https://www.aboutibs.org/low-fodmap-diet/measuring-fodmaps-in-foods.html